The Way Mum Does It

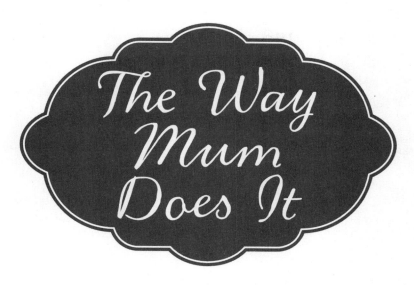

The Way Mum Does It

Treasured family advice
from Australian mothers

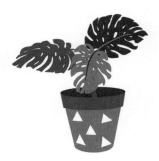

*More than 400 pearls of wisdom
shared by the Over60 online community*

Edited by Alexandra O'Brien

ABC
Books

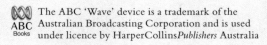 The ABC 'Wave' device is a trademark of the Australian Broadcasting Corporation and is used under licence by HarperCollins*Publishers* Australia

First published in Australia in 2018
by HarperCollins*Publishers* Australia Pty Limited
ABN 36 009 913 517
harpercollins.com.au

Compilation copyright © The Seniors Ad Network Pty Ltd 2018

HarperCollins*Publishers*
Level 13, 201 Elizabeth Street, Sydney NSW 2000, Australia
Unit D1, 63 Apollo Drive, Rosedale, Auckland 0632, New Zealand
A 53, Sector 57, Noida, UP, India
1 London Bridge Street, London, SE1 9GF, United Kingdom
2 Bloor Street East, 20th floor, Toronto, Ontario M4W 1A8, Canada
195 Broadway, New York NY 10007, USA

National Library of Australia Cataloguing-in-Publication entry:

The way mum does it : treasured family advice from
Australian mothers / edited by Alexandra O'Brien
ISBN: 978 0 7333 3840 3 (paperback)
ISBN: 978 1 4607 0839 2 (ebook)
Includes index.
Home economics—Miscellanea.
Health—Miscellanea.
Gardening--Miscellanea.
Travel—Miscellanea.
Mothers—Australia.
O'Brien, Alexandra, editor.

Cover design and internal design by Hazel Lam, HarperCollins Design Studio
Cover and internal images by shutterstock.com
Printed and bound in Australia by McPhersons Printing Group
The papers used by HarperCollins in the manufacture of this book are a natural, recyclable product made from wood grown in sustainable plantation forests. The fibre source and manufacturing processes meet recognised international environmental standards, and carry certification.

Dedicated to mums everywhere,
who recognise the importance of
passing on their wisdom, so it can be
treasured for generations to come.

Contents

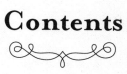

Introduction

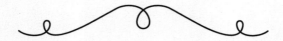

'To describe my mother would be to write about a hurricane in its perfect power. Or the climbing, falling colours of a rainbow.'

— *Maya Angelou, American poet, author and activist*

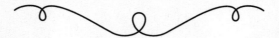

There's not a fitting description that sufficiently captures the sheer importance of what mothers (and fathers, for that matter) do. Likewise, it's a mean feat to put into words what mothers mean to their families. Try as we might (as teenagers who know it all) *not* to become our mothers as we grow up, I think it's fair to say we all reach a point in life when the weight of what our mothers have done for us hits us, and a newfound sense of understanding, appreciation and love prevails. You might go as far as to say that, in some ways, mothers are akin to superheroes – they're there when you need them (and even when you don't know you need them), they seem to have a solution to everything (no matter how big or small the problem), they can always make you feel better, they teach you endless things about the world (and yourself) and, no matter what, they will always be there (maybe just in memory and spirit) to support and encourage you.

I am fortunate enough to say this is true of my mother, Cheryl, who simultaneously raised five daughters, kept an immaculate home, cooked beautiful food and hosted perfect dinners, all while taking the time to care for the different personalities of her children, providing unwavering care and support. She helped my sisters and me become the people we are today. It's also no surprise that she is now doing the exact same thing for her six grandchildren. I know there are many versions of this story. And it's not just mums. Dads are wonderful, too – in some cases, Dad takes the place of Mum.

There comes the day when we all need to grow up and fly the nest, so to speak. Or, God forbid, the day when – due to circumstance, geography or, sadly, death – our mothers simply are not around. To make this reality more bearable, we wanted to chronicle all the pearls of wisdom from mothers in one place. Think of this as a manual of the best advice from mothers across Australia, which can be passed on for generations to come.

You can't bottle a mother's encouraging words, priceless hugs or helpful actions, but we hope this comes close.

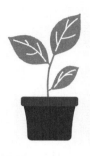

Life

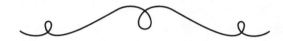

'My mother always said, "You can't have it all!" When I was young, I set out to prove her wrong. She was, of course, right.'

— Noni Hazlehurst, Australian actress, director, writer, presenter and broadcaster

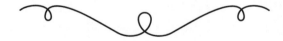

The best thing my mother ever taught me: when something tragic or unexpected happens in life, from personal disasters to chipping a nail, don't dwell on it. Pick yourself up, dust yourself off and get on with it. Start remedying it. Put the practical necessities in place first, then deal with the rest as it comes. Look at what positives there are, however small.

'This was how my mother and father lived their lives. They had a big family with little money and it was the only way to live. They couldn't give up, or get help. They had to deal with what life threw at them and survive. That is it really, how to survive. I am forever grateful for being taught this.' – *Therese Webb*

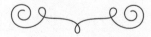

Remember, this too shall pass.

'My mother experienced periods of depression and when I also showed signs of it, she took me aside one day and very quietly said, "Remember the other day when things were good and you were happy? That ended, and so will this."' – *Susan Kelly*

You must have a good bed and a good pair of shoes. If you are not in one you are in the other.

'This tip came from my mother when I was about to get married (47 years ago). I heard it repeated frequently when anyone was going to buy boots, shoes or beds.' – *Lorraine Phillips*

Tip 1: Never trouble trouble until trouble troubles you; it's always double trouble and troubles others, too.

Tip 2: A friend is not a fellow who is taken in by sham; a friend is one who knows our faults and doesn't give a damn.

'My tip is actually two sayings that were hung on our dining room wall; I have followed them all my life. My mother passed these sayings on to her three children. She was a very down-to-earth person who was loved by all the neighbourhood.' – *Barbara Kelly*

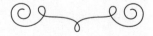

Never change the bed linen on Fridays. Never put new shoes on the table. Never cross your knife and fork. Never walk under a ladder. All of these will cause bad luck. And, if you spill the salt, always take a pinch and throw it over your shoulder for good luck.

'My mother always said these things to me growing up and I say them to my kids. Who of course just roll their eyes.' – *Lee Quine*

Live for today because tomorrow may never come. – *Maureen Farrell*

How to be on time, every time

Do you struggle to be on time? For countless years, mothers have stressed to their children how important it is to be on time. Here are four time-tested tips passed down from mothers over the years to ensure you're right on time, all of the time.

1. Don't set yourself up to fail

If you know that you drag the chain in the morning and find it hard to get moving, then a 7.30 a.m. breakfast catch-up is not something you want to schedule. Rather than agreeing to a meeting or social engagement first thing, suggest a time that suits you, on a day that you know you will have time to get there.

2. Prepare as much as you can

When you've got to be up and out the door – to get to the airport or a gym class, for example – you don't have time to be searching for a lost shoe. Set out your clothes the night before, and pack everything you need in a bag (and leave it by the front door). This will make your morning much less stressful.

3. Assume the worst

Depending where you have to be, always allow 'buffer time' to deal with unexpected delays. Things like traffic, broken lifts or empty petrol tanks can throw a spanner in the works – so allow for them when making your travel plans.

4. Use online tools

If you're going somewhere you haven't been to before, nowadays there are lots of online resources to help. Always check an online map first to see how long they estimate it will take. Then add your extra buffer time on top. You can also use the calendar on your phone or computer to schedule your appointments with reminders. This way you can avoid double-booking yourself.

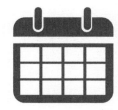

Never put all your eggs in one basket.

'I think this refers to all things in life. That we take each day as it comes, make the right decisions, be thankful, honour one another and share with others.' – *Elizabeth Rooney*

Better cobwebs on the ceiling than cobwebs on the mind.

'My mother and I were great readers and sometimes felt guilty about our lack of enthusiasm for housework. Mum would trot out this saying to ease our guilt. It worked well for me.' – *Shirley Bannear*

It's not the dead ones you want to be scared of;
it's the live ones.

'As a child, Mum and Dad would take me to the
cemetery and I was always scared. Mum would always
say this to me. I think this was her best life and
parenting tip. Thank you, Mum.' – *Sue Moppett*

You need two lives. The first one is an experiment;
the second one is to get it right.

'It came from my mother-in-law, who was like a
mum to me.' – *Deborah Walsh*

3 ways to boost your motivation

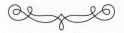

When you feel unmotivated it can be tough to get things done. Even simple tasks can feel like a burden. So if your 'get up and go' has got up and gone, follow our tips below to help you get it back.

1. Remember how you feel in the moment

Sometimes the task on our mental to-do list looks just plain boring and we don't want to do it. But often, when we are in the moment (or have finished it), we can feel a real sense of accomplishment. For instance, you might dread sending off your invoice for the consulting work you do. It seems like so much effort to gather all of your paperwork together. But what about that great feeling when your pay packet lands in your account? Remember the positive aspects of your task (which can be hard when you have 99 other things on your to-do list); this can help push you to get it done.

2. Play the 'so that' game

Sometimes when you're in the trenches it can be hard to see what you're doing has meaning, or is worthwhile. Try this simple trick. Say to yourself, 'I need to do this task so that ...' and fill in the reason. For instance: 'I need to pack away the laundry so that my room feels comfortable and relaxing before I go to bed.' Or: 'I need to finish this report so that I can get paid enough money to support my family.' This helps you zero in on why you need to do what you do.

3. Do it your way

Sometimes there is a more fun way to complete a task. For example, you might hate mopping, but what if you could do it while you blast music from the stereo and have a dance around at the same time? You might be worried about a speech you need to write, but what if you could write it in a room with a sea view, cold drink in hand? Now that sounds pretty good, doesn't it?

Don't wait for a girl to find out you're a slob in the bedroom.

'This was advice from a mum to her son (me) rather than a daughter, but very sage advice it was. I was a 17-year-old still at home and, like most, a real mess in my room. Never put anything away, clothes on the floor, bed never made, and so on. Mum tried many things to get me to clean my room, but finally said that no girl would want to spend a night in my room unless I kept it tidy. From that day on, I tried to do better in the tidy room department – and I think that she was right.' – *Alan Evans*

Careful of your tongue, it's in a wet place and is likely to slip. – *Shona Campbell*

Your life spreads before you like a carpet of snow; be careful where you tread for every step will show.

'My mum wrote this in my autograph book many years ago and I've never forgotten it. My dear mum is 93 now and in a nursing home.' – *Glynis Scotland*

Stay focused and when you do something, make sure you give it 100 per cent.

'This came from my gorgeous 87-year-old mum, who was always so proud of me because I was really good at school. She regrets that I was not able to go further with my studies because we were busy with a family of eight children. I was the oldest girl and helped out a lot with the younger ones. To this day, she often asks me if I blame her. No way, she was a fantastic mum and did what she could. Now I only live 15 kilometres away from her and my only remaining brother is her carer. She has buried five of her children and raised two grandchildren from the ages of four and six – they are now in their thirties.' – *Shirley Whitehouse*

9 habits that will make you happier

This sage advice mothers and grandmothers having been sharing for years has now been backed up by research. Yet another reason to get working on turning that frown upside down.

1. Keep a gratitude journal
Recording the things you're grateful for can have a potent impact on your mood.

2. Get awestruck
The emotion of awe can have a powerful impact on your stress levels and boost feelings of contentment.

3. Meditate
You've heard it before no doubt, but meditation works! Regular meditation, even in short bursts, can help improve your mood.

4. Get outside
Wide-open spaces are a powerful tonic for frayed nerves and a racing mind. Whether it's a forest, park, beach or lake, get outside – disconnect from the modern world and reconnect with the natural world. Your mind will thank you for it.

5. Do the things you do when you're happy, even if you're not

Positive emotions have the power to neutralise negative ones. Taking part in activities you do when you're happy can help trigger the emotions you usually experience when you're feeling good, helping to shift the blues.

6. Volunteer

While it might sound daunting, especially when you're feeling low, helping others can be the best way to help yourself. Studies have backed up what Mother knew – volunteering is linked with a reduced risk of depression and higher levels of satisfaction.

7. Be social

Spending time with friends and family is one of the best ways to neutralise a low mood.

8. Get your hands dirty

Not only can gardening offer plenty of health and wellness benefits, it can also lift your spirits directly, thanks to bacteria commonly found in soil! The harmless *Mycobacterium vaccae* bacterium can stimulate the release of serotonin in the brain. Low serotonin levels can be a cause of depression.

9. Exercise

Whether it's walking or swimming, hiking or a step class, regular exercise is one of the best ways to maintain a sense of wellbeing. Mum used to always tell you to run outside and play; now research has shown that just 20 minutes of exercise can boost your mood.

Invite widows or widowers to your home to share a special dinner or BBQ throughout the festive season. There are a lot of lonely people who have no family around them at this special time of the year.

'My grandmother, who died some 60 years ago, shared this kindness with me. It has stuck with me and lifts me up.' – *Des Howell*

Silence is golden.

'Don't just blurt things out to someone; give it some thought before you go to say something that might affect you later. Sometimes it's better to say nothing at all.' – *Shannon Shepherdson*

Never chase after boys or trams. There's always another one along in a little while!

'My tip to my daughters and granddaughters.'
— *Brenda Carter*

My mum would say that you could always tell a person by their shoes. — *Wendy Vincent*

Don't start anything unless you can finish it.

'As the youngest of 14 it was wise advice: don't pick a fight, start an argument or a job to do unless you can complete it. In a busy family no one has time to clean up your messes. Saved a lot of angst, too.'
— *Maureen Petzel*

There is so much good in the worst of us, and so much bad in the best of us, that it does not behove any of us to talk about the rest of us.

'My mum lived to be 100. I cared for her for many years; this was one of her favourite sayings and she taught it to me when I was young. My mum never had any family – her parents, brothers and sister all died in Dublin of the Spanish flu, which meant she fended for herself. I was her only child. Unmarried, Catholic and Irish, her life was not easy, but she worked until she was 78. She got cancer and went through all the usual things. As she got older and older, I had to do more and more. I miss her. This was one of her favourite sayings – one, I might add, that she did not always adhere to.' – *Catherina North*

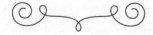

You will catch more flies with honey than vinegar.

'Her advice still endures 50 years on. It has enabled me to enjoy my life being the people-person my mother was. Way more than "catching flies", it's a standard of kindness when dealing with others. With the softer "honey" approach, tempers and negativity are soothed and not inflamed, as a lashing of vinegar invariably causes. The roll-on effect is that it's far easier to be kind to oneself with a habit of kindness to others – especially in difficult or volatile situations. Her words became the model of behaviour I learned to live by. I can't imagine living life without her words of wisdom. Thank God for mothers, mine especially!' – *Maggie Skinner*

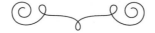

Always wear good undies because you never know if you might have a fall or end up at the doctor's or in hospital.

'My mother always told my sister and me this. My sister is only 11 months younger than I am so we did everything together. Mum made identical clothes for us so we were always dressed the same, sometimes just different colours. My mum sewed all of our clothes – even our school uniforms – and hand-knitted my jumpers. My clothes were beautiful, some with applique. I longed to just go to the shops and buy something off a rack. She also was a great home cook and we always had homemade jams and puddings. She was famous for her apple pies and caramel tarts. Now, my mother is in a home with Alzheimer's; I long for one of her homemade garments and apple pies.' – *Deslee Till*

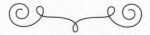

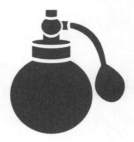

Beauty and health

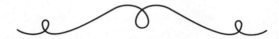

'Advice my mother gave to me: "Brush your eyebrows every night. Why? To give them a good shape. Sometimes putting a little Vaseline on them is beneficial. Don't forget to moisturise your neck every night using upward strokes. Necks need all the help they can get."'

— *Ita Buttrose, AO OBE, Australian media icon and businesswoman*

These tips are for general advice only and should not be relied on as health advice. Before trying a new health remedy, you should consider seeking advice from a doctor or qualified health practitioner.

Beauty Tips

For beautiful hands, whenever you are in the sun, remember to apply sunscreen to the backs of your hands, too. The sun does a lot of damage to this area and can make your hands looked aged. A lot of people don't think to do this.

'I was admiring my mum's beautiful hands and made a comment about how nice they looked. She said to me, "Annette, the best bit of advice I can give you to look youthful is to apply sunscreen to the back of your hands whenever you are in the sun." I have always remembered this and I have now passed it on to my daughter, whom I hope will follow this simple but effective tip.' – *Annette Draper*

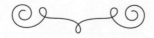

Never ever go to bed with your make-up on. Always use a moisturiser on your skin – whatever you can afford. It's not about the price; it's about what suits you. Always cover your skin when out in the sun. A hat, an umbrella, long sleeves or just simply stay out of it.

'My mother sadly passed away in her 98th year, three years ago. There are so many legacies that she gave me to remember forever, whether it be cooking, cleaning or tips on parenting – the most important being how to care for my skin. My earliest memory was of the product that she used: Ponds Vanishing Cream, in a white jar with a pink lid. My mum, Violet, came from a harsh background, as many did from that era. Her father made her and her three brothers work hard on their property in the harsh Australian sun. Mum's skin was beautiful; she never ever looked her age. If she was asked, most people were shocked by her answer.' – *Lynette Johnston*

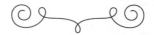

From around the age of 11 or 12, start wearing moisturiser on your face and neck every morning, to help prevent wrinkles as you get older.

'Mum always used a cream on her face every morning and being the oldest girl I asked her why. "It helps to keep my wrinkles away," she used to say to me. When I was a teenager people used to think my mum was my older sister. And when Mum passed away at the age of 90, she didn't look her age. I am nearly 70 and I think it works for me. I have passed the tip down to my daughter and my granddaughter. Thank you, Mum.' – *Marlene Marguerite Poletti*

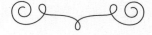

Clean and moisturise your skin everyday!
No need for expensive brands.

'From my mum as soon as I started using
make-up. My mum always had beautiful skin.'
— *Catherine Christie*

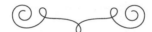

Make your own moisturiser

Using 30 ml almond, jojoba or argan oil as the base, add
a few drops essential oils (such as rose geranium, carrot
seed, lavender, chamomile, rosemary or lemongrass).
Far from making your skin feel greasy, oils absorb
rapidly into the skin. You can also use coconut oil, but
note that this is solid at room temperature so it will
need to be warmed before blending. The antimicrobial
properties of coconut oil can be beneficial to those with
problematic skin such as acne and imperfections.

The dos and don'ts of daring lip colour

Watching your mother apply lipstick when you were young is more than just a fond memory; it's a beauty lesson. A sharp contrast between your lip colour and your complexion can help you look younger. But how do you wear a bold lipstick without it bleeding, smudging onto your teeth or needing constant reapplication? It's easier than you think. Collected from many a mother, this is the ultimate list of dos and don'ts for wearing a bold-coloured lipstick.

Do: Be prepared
Exfoliate your lips first with an exfoliating cream, or just a toothbrush and a smear of Vaseline or lip balm. This will help prevent your colour from clumping together over dry cracked lips.

Do: Consider lip liner
There's a reason your mother – and grandmother before her – were partial to lip liner. Liner will help your colour last longer and make it look more defined. To create a steady line around your lips, look in the mirror and smile with your mouth closed so the lips are perfectly taut.

Do: Use a lip brush
Using a good-quality lip brush will prevent you from accidentally over-applying, which is the main cause of lipstick

bleeding into fine lines around the mouth and it rubbing off on teeth. Start at the centre of your lower lip, moving out to the corners. Press lips together, then apply on your upper lip starting at the cupid's bow.

Don't: Be afraid!

Choosing the right shade and finish for you is a game of trial and error. In general, berry pinks, fuchsias or anything with cooler, blue undertones will make your teeth look whiter, whereas scarlet reds, bright oranges and colours with warmer undertones can make your teeth look yellow. Go to a make-up counter to get some personalised advice. Remember, if you hate it, wipe it off and start again. That's the worst that can happen!

Don't: Layer on applications

When your lip colour fades, avoid the temptation to add more on top as this could lead to build-up and clumping. Instead, wipe off the old application and start again with a fresh coat.

Don't: Overdo it

If you're going to brave a bold new lip colour, keep the rest of your look natural. Avoid too much eyeliner and keep your blush soft so that your mouth, literally, does all the talking!

Don't: Go overboard

Watch what you're wearing. For example, don't wear red lips with a purple top unless you're feeling eccentric, and don't overdo your jewellery. Teaming bold lipstick with black, white and neutral shades, plus simple accessories, will make a modern statement.

Always put your lippy on when going out or having visitors over.

'My mother was a lady and always dressed well. Whenever we were going out, Mum would always come up with this one-liner. I've never forgotten this good advice. We miss her.' – *Nanette Smith*

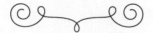

When applying lipstick, an easy way to ensure your lipstick doesn't rub off on your teeth is to wash your hands with soap, pop an index finger just under your lips and close your lips over your finger. Once you've applied your lippie, pop your finger in then draw it out. Any errant lippy will come away with your finger.

'When my friend's mother taught me this trick, it was a game changer for me. No more worrying about a lipstick-smeared smile!' – *Jessie Lee*

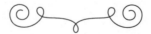

4 home remedies
for split ends

Remember the days when grandmothers reminded their granddaughters to brush their hair 100 strokes a day? Well, if you were lucky enough for Grandma to do the brushing for you, then it would have been a very relaxing experience.

While keeping your hair soft and knot-free is important, so is getting rid of split ends. Home hair treatments for split ends can be a great help, too, because they don't cost you an arm and a leg, you often already have everything you need in your kitchen, and you can use these methods again and again.

1. Castor oil
Simply mix together equal amounts of castor oil, mustard oil and olive oil. The amount you use will depend on how thick your hair is. All you have to do is apply the mixture into your hair, wrap it up in a towel and let it set for 30 minutes. Then simply wash your hair as normal and comb.

2. Honey

Honey is great as a home hair treatment for split ends, especially when you mix it with yogurt. All you need is a half-cup of yogurt and a tablespoon of honey, mixed together well. Massage into your hair, paying particular attention to the ends, and leave in for 20 minutes. When you rinse it off, just use water.

3. Beer

This is a bit of an odd one, but people swear by the beer hair treatment – and it's so easy. Simply grab some beer, pour it through your hair and wait for it to dry. No mixing or stirring necessary! Wash and condition as normal afterwards.

4. Avocado

If you eat a lot of avocado, you may have noticed that your hair and skin become extremely soft. To take it up a notch, all you have to do is mash up an avocado and, after dampening your hair, massage the fruit into your hair. Make sure you get your split ends coated. Let it set for anywhere between 15 and 30 minutes, then rinse it out. This is a great way to use avocados that are on the turn so they don't go to waste!

For a natural way to set waves or curls in your hair, dissolve sugar in warm water and comb through hair before using curlers or pins. When dry, the curl should stay in and smell sweet.
If going on a date, add a drop of perfume or essential oil to the water.

'My grandmother passed this on to my mother when she was a child and they set her hair in pin curls. My mother used it on my hair for ballet concerts when I needed a tight bun or a curled ponytail. Then I did the same for my daughters. Now my granddaughter has her gymnastics and dancing hairstyles styled the same way by her natural and organic-focused mum.'
– Karen Howell

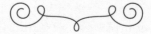

How to banish the green chlorine tinge from hair!

Here's a trick for banishing the 'chlorine green' from your hair in summertime. The greenish tinge in your hair actually comes from trace amounts of copper in the water, but the chlorine assists in fixing it to your hair.

Mix a palmful of bicarbonate of soda with your regular shampoo, then scrub through your hair and leave in for a few minutes. Rinse thoroughly, then condition your hair as normal.

To help stop the chlorine and copper attacking your hair in the first place, wet your hair before going in the pool and use a swimming cap. (Yes, the one Mother always insisted you wear!) You can also comb leave-in conditioner through your hair before donning the cap, if your hair is especially prone to going green.

4 ways to create volume in your hair

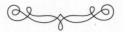

From rags to hot curlers, and from curling irons to crimpers, women have turned to all manner of tools over the years in the quest of voluminous locks. Sometimes, however, instead of spending lots of money on the latest hair styling tool on the market, some old-fashioned tips are just the ticket. Here are four simple ways to combat flat hair at home.

1. Cut back on washing

Washing your hair only once or twice a week should be sufficient for most hair types. This may seem strange since hair tends to be the lankest when it's oily, but if you over-wash your hair, you strip it of essential oils that keep it healthy and lifted.

2. Wash with bicarbonate of soda

When you do wash your hair, use one part bicarb soda and three parts water. It clarifies and adds volume to your hair by removing the build up from dirt, shampoo and conditioner that could be weighing down your roots.

3. Change your part

Never let your hair get used to a part, this can lead to cowlicks and even hair thinning. Switch up your part every morning to help keep your roots lifted, or, simply wear a different hairstyle.

4. Blow dry upside down

Let gravity take its natural path and blow dry your hair from the roots down while it is flipped away from the scalp. Use a light hairspray that you find works for you, but wait 30 seconds after spraying it before you stand up straight again. This is how long hairspray takes to set.

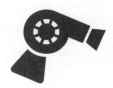

2 easy DIY face treatments

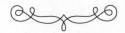

Forget expensive salon treatments for your beauty fix. Your mum would want you to save your pennies for a rainy day with these do-at-home face masks.

Treatment 1: Baking powder to get glowing

For a quick collagen-boosting, brightening-and-tightening face treatment, look no further than your pantry. Say hello to baking powder – a saviour that mothers have been turning to for generations for a host of uses. Not only is it great for circulation, it has clarifying properties that help your skin glow.

You will need:

1 tablespoon water

1 tablespoon baking powder

1 teaspoon honey

How to:

In a clean bowl, combine ingredients and mix into a paste. Using a clean spoon, apply a thick layer over the face, working your way down to the neck. Relax for 5 minutes.

Using a face washer and warm water, gently pat mixture off face. Follow treatment with your normal moisturising routine.

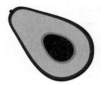

Treatment 2: Avocado rescue for lacklustre skin

If you suffer from dry skin, you're not alone. Whether it's the harsh environment outdoors, or the constant heating or air conditioning indoors, our skin is taken from one extreme to the other almost every day. As a result, skin can be quite lacklustre. Fear not, this lovely mask is nourishing, creamy and has soothing properties by way of Greek yogurt.

You will need:

1/2 avocado, mashed

1 tablespoon plain or Greek yogurt
   (avoid using Greek-style yogurts)

How to:

In a clean bowl, combine ingredients. Using a clean spoon, apply a thick layer over the face. Relax for 20 minutes.

Pat mask off using a face washer and warm water, and follow with your normal moisturising routine.

8 natural dandruff remedies from your pantry

There's no need to spend your cash on anti-dandruff shampoo when there's a solution hiding in the pantry.

1. Tea tree oil

A lot of anti-dandruff treatments contain tea tree oil, and with good reason. This oil can help reduce the flaking and itchiness of dandruff, so just add a capful to your regular shampoo bottle.

2. Aloe vera

It's not just for sunburn! You can rub aloe vera from a plant or pure aloe vera gel in a tube onto wet hair to relieve the itchy scalp that often accompanies dandruff. Then wash your hair as normal.

3. Olive oil

Just like the old home-remedy treatment for a baby's cradle cap, olive oil can help sooth a dandruff-prone scalp, too. Wet your hair and warm the oil a little bit first. Rub in the oil, massaging the scalp, and wrap hair in a towel or shower cap. Leave for at least 30 minutes, then rinse out with a mild shampoo.

4. Salt

Yes, really. The grains of salt will act as a scrub to help remove dry skin from your scalp. Apply a handful of salt to wet hair and give it a good scrub with your fingertips before rinsing well.

5. Apple cider vinegar

Not just for salad dressing, this vinegar is great at fixing up the pH balance of your hair, which can cause the itch. Simply mix 1/3 cup apple cider vinegar with the same amount of water. Pour onto your wet hair, rub in and leave for 5 minutes to soak before rinsing well.

6. Lemon juice

Fresh lemon juice is a nice-smelling treatment. Rub onto wet hair, then allow it to sit for a couple of minutes before washing out. Best to avoid this one if your skin is sensitive as the acidic juice might sting.

7. Bicarb soda

Is there anything this stuff can't do? Add a 1/4 cup baking soda to a cupful of warm water and mix well. Then rub into wet hair, scrub and rinse off.

8. Coconut oil

Another pantry staple with so many uses. This remedy not only smells good, it helps to put back the natural oils that your hair needs when suffering from dandruff. Rub the oil into your hands and then apply to damp hair. Try to leave in for at least 30 minutes before washing out.

Clear a case of cradle cap

Cradle cap is a mild condition caused when a baby's scalp produces too much sebum. Flaky or oily crusts appear across the scalp, and sometimes elsewhere on the body. While cradle cap often clears up on its own, you can gently soften the crusts by massaging coconut or olive oil into your baby's scalp after their bath. Leave overnight, then wash your baby's hair with mild baby shampoo the following morning and use a soft brush to help loosen the flakes. Never pick at them. Repeat daily until the head is free of crusting.

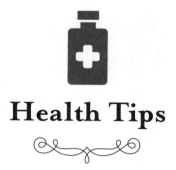

Health Tips

Use lavender, cloves and mint in water for freshness, wounds, pain, skin problems, mild burns, cleaning, calmness and wellness. Use essential oils for arthritis and asthma, hay fever and sinus – as well as a home and car freshener.

'This has been passed down to me by my nanna, who was from Cyprus and then lived in Egypt. That is where she met my pop, an Australian soldier in the First World War. Nanna, of course, learnt about the essential oils and water from her mother, who was Syrian born.' – *Karen Boyd*

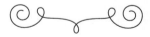

Herbal remedies that have stood the test of time

For years, mothers and grandmothers have been passing along their secrets to solve a number of health concerns. These remedies have stood the test of time. While these should never replace consulting your doctor, it doesn't hurt to also try the natural option as well.

Problem: Poor quality of sleep
Try … chamomile. It contains a range of components with anti-stress properties. Either opt for an organic chamomile tea or buy the dried flowers. Add 2 teaspoons flowers to 100 ml water. Cover and steep for 3 minutes. The reason it's good to cover the water is that the active compounds are in the essential oils, which can dissipate if exposed.

Problem: Upset stomach
Try … ginger. With antispasmodic and anti-nausea properties, people have been using ginger to curb nausea and vomiting for years. Try a teaspoon of grated ginger in hot water and be sure not to make it too weak, as you will miss out on its therapeutic benefits.

Problem: Tension headache

Try ... magnesium. If you're suffering from a tension headache, you could be lacking magnesium. Available as a supplement as magnesium oxide, the common dosage is 400–500 mg per day. Check with your doctor first, however, if you are taking medications that may be contraindicated. To add magnesium to your diet, opt for kale and spinach, or pumpkin seeds, almonds or (hooray!) dark chocolate.

Also, using aromatherapy oils is another great way to ease a sore head. Into 2 teaspoons carrier oil (such as almond or jojoba), add 2 drops each rosemary, lemongrass or lavender oil. Rub into the nape of the neck and temples.

Problem: Low energy

Try ... acai berry. Talked about a lot recently as a superfood, the power-packed Amazon acai berry can boost your energy. Really great for busy people, try it in powdered form either added to a juice or on cereal, or in a capsule. Follow the packet directions for the recommended dose – in powdered form, this is usually 1000 mg.

Problem: Feeling stressed

Try ... withania. As most of us are multi-tasking at a million miles an hour, our adrenal glands can get exhausted. That's when we burn out and get run down. Used in Indian Ayurvedic medicine, this herb can help to look after the nervous system and the adrenals.

Withania (also called Indian ginseng or ashwagandha) is available in tablet form. Follow the dosage directions on the bottle, or take advice from your dispensing practitioner.

Alternatively, try this traditional Ayurvedic recipe:
Heat I teaspoon ground withania root and 1–2 teaspoons honey in 1½ cups milk (or milk and water). Simmer gently for 10–15 minutes, until mixture has reduced by 1/3, then remove from heat, strain and drink before bed. Optional: add a pinch of black pepper and/or cinnamon to the withania mixture before cooking.

Problem: Eczema

Try … calendula. An extract of this marigold-like flower is commonly used in skin lotions. Eczema sufferers have turned to calendula ointments because of its purported skin-healing properties; it can also help to reduce pain and inflammation. You can find calendula products, such as soaps, oils and lotions, at health food stores.

Your grandmother may have made her own stove-top preparation, using fresh calendula flowers from her garden. Lightly crush 15 g fresh calendula flowers and heat with 1/3 cup (80 ml) coconut or olive oil in a double boiler over very low heat for 2 hours. Strain into a very clean jar, pressing flowers with the back of a spoon to release all the oils and allow to cool before using. Keep in fridge.

My mum said I should never go to bed on an empty stomach full of beer.

'This was typical of my mum, who was always concerned that I had enough to eat. When you're a teenager, though, thinking about food was far from my thoughts!' – *Clive Tudge*

Use evaporated milk on sunburn to draw the heat out of the burn.

'My aunt was very fair-skinned and the very first time she went to the beach she was badly sunburned. My grandmother applied evaporated milk on her sunburn and it would draw the heat out of the burn. The evaporated milk would then dry and crack and Granny would wash it off with a cold wet cloth and reapply. It actually healed the sunburn quickly. I was there while my granny was applying the evaporated milk, at the same time telling my aunt she could never go to the beach again. This was way before we knew about sunscreen.' – *Linda English*

To help a cut or bruise on the body, wait for it to heal and then apply coconut oil to the area to help reduce scarring.

'As a child, I used to get a lot of cuts and bruises. My mum's coconut oil trick helped with the healing process.' – *Vince Misquitta*

Thistle milk to remove warts.

'Grandmother used to take me into the garden of an evening and apply the milk of thistle weed on the wart on my finger. With continuing application, presto! The wart was gone. Love my grandma. I guess I was about five years old, but still remember the miracle of the disappearing wart.' – *Fay Barker*

8 alternative uses for mouthwash

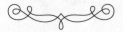

You'll be pleased to know that your humble mouthwash could actually be working much harder for you around the house. It's a great multi-purpose product that's ideal for travelling or just saving space in the medicine cabinet at home.

1. Stop the itch

If you're camping and find yourself being eaten alive by mosquitoes, pull out the mouthwash. Apply to the affected area to relieve the itch and sting. You can also use mouthwash on your hair if you have an itchy, flaky scalp. Just mix equal parts water and mouthwash and apply it to your hair post-shampoo, before rinsing and conditioning.

2. Keep flowers happy

Add a capful of mouthwash to the vase water and this will help keep the bacteria at bay that cause flowers to die too soon.

3. Clean your hands

If you are out and about without access to soap and water, you can use mouthwash as a stand-in for hand sanitiser. You can also use it to get rid of odours on your skin, such as onion or garlic, after cooking.

4. Protect plants

If you want to save an indoor plant from fungus or mould, spray it with a combination of 1/4 mouthwash and 3/4 water.

5. Clean a mirror

Run out of glass cleaner? Use mouthwash in the same way for brilliant results.

6. Clean a cut

The alcohol in mouthwash makes it ideal to clean a cut before you cover it with a Bandaid. You can also use mouthwash for cleaning infected piercings, ingrown toenails or even pimples.

7. Treat foot fungus

Add some mouthwash to a tub of warm water and soak affected feet for 45+ minutes before rinsing. You can also add mouthwash to trainers that have been in contact with athlete's foot.

8. Deodorant

If you get stuck, you can use mouthwash as deodorant as it will fight bacteria under your arms (as well as in your mouth). If your skin is sensitive or freshly shaved, however, this is best avoided.

How to fall asleep in less than a minute

For generations, mothers have been sharing their wisdom on the importance of sleep. However, try as you might to get a good night's shut-eye, sometimes falling asleep just isn't that easy. Without a doubt, this trick is going to leave a lot of people skeptical but don't knock it till you try it ... it really does work. After all, if you have experienced many a sleepless night, what have you go to lose?

It's called the '4–7–8' breathing technique. The short explanation: you breathe in through your nose for 4 seconds, hold your breath for 7 seconds and exhale through your mouth for 8 seconds. It isn't just a random selection of numbers, either; this studied combination has now widely been reported to have a chemical-like effect on the brain – it slows your heart rate and soothes you to sleep.

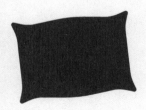

What it does:

By extending your inhale to a count of 4, you are forcing yourself to take in more oxygen. By holding your breath for 7 seconds, you allow the oxygen to affect your bloodstream. By exhaling steadily for 8 seconds, you then emit carbon dioxide from your lungs.

In order to hold your breath for 7 seconds and then to exhale for 8, your body is forced to slow your heart rate. You can immediately feel your heart rate slow down, your mind become quieter, and your whole body relax.

It will instantly relax your heart, mind and overall central nervous system. The technique has an almost sedative drug-like effect for some people.

Our verdict:

Free, easy and works in an instant – what's not to love? From using 4–7–8 to get back to sleep if you wake in the night, to having a go-to exercise to calm frayed nerves, there's a reason everyone is talking about this how-to-fall-asleep-in-less-than-a-minute trick.

Natural ways to boost your vitamin D

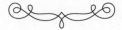

Known as the 'sunshine vitamin', maintaining the right level of vitamin D is essential to keep you healthy. Luckily, there are a number of ways you can naturally boost your intake.

Apart from bone health, vitamin D is also linked to many other functions in the body. We've done the legwork for you. It's beneficial for cardiovascular health, rheumatoid arthritis, cancer, glucose intolerance, multiple sclerosis, type 1 and type 2 diabetes, depression and protection against colds. Here are four ways you can ensure adequate intake – and naturally, too! But, like most things in life, a combination of diet, supplements and environment is the key.

Sunlight

The best source of vitamin D is UV-B radiation from the sun. Approximately 5 to 30 minutes of sun exposure while not wearing sunscreen (between 10 a.m. and 3 p.m.), at least twice a week, will do the job.

It is worth keeping in mind that UV radiation levels vary depending on your location, time of year and time of day, so make sure you wear sun protection when the UV Index is 3 or above. In some states, UV radiation is higher and you need sun protection all year round at certain times of the day. Cancer Council Australia says that, for most people, adequate vitamin D levels are reached through regular daily activity and incidental exposure to the sun.

To check UV levels and the times sun protection is required, look on the Bureau of Meteorology website at www.bom.gov.au – search for 'UV and sun protection services'.

Diet

You can incorporate many food options into your diet to make sure you have healthy levels of the sunshine vitamin. Think fatty fish (sardines, herring, mackerel, tuna and salmon), canned tuna, milk fortified with vitamin D, egg yolks and cereals fortified with vitamin D.

Supplements

From tablets and capsules to liquids, supplements are a convenient way to ensure you are getting enough vitamin D. Even better: There are natural supplement options available. Be careful, though, as too much can be toxic. Depending on your situation, daily dosages vary. Consult your doctor to find out what's best for you.

Cod liver oil

If you're not a fan of fatty fish, then you'll be pleased to know that cod liver oil – which comes from the liver of the cod fish – is rich in vitamins A and D. You can either buy it in liquid or capsule form; check the bottle for daily dose recommendations and consult your doctor to find out what the best dosage is for you.

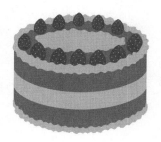

Cooking

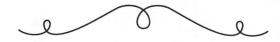

'Eat well but don't overeat! You can eat anything you feel like in moderation, as long it makes you happy.'

—Angie Hong, style icon, former restaurateur and chef Dan Hong's mum

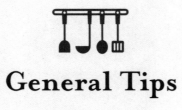

General Tips

We always grew our own vegetables growing up, so when we said we were hungry, the saltshaker was handed out the door and we were told to go and help ourselves in the garden. We always had tomatoes, peas, radishes and carrots.

'Mum always wanted us to eat good food, and special treats were given on baking day on Saturday. I still love my veggies! I learnt from an early age to tend the garden beds, and knew where my food came from.' – *Kim Cardiff*

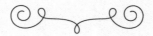

To check if your eggs are fresh, fill a basin with water – a fresh egg will lie flat on the bottom, a not-so-fresh egg will rise slightly and a bad egg will float to the top.

'My mum is 85 years old and always loved chooks. She used to spoil them with all fresh produce that was grown from our garden. When they stopped producing eggs she'd cut their heads off. After plucking and cleaning them, she'd cook them in the pressure cooker with curry and vegetables. I never tasted a roasted chicken until I was older.'
– *Janice Fanias*

If you're running late cooking tea, simply set the table as though it looks like you're on time. It's just that the food isn't.

'Dad always got home from the pub at six. Mum was always involved in local community activities and we would arrive home just before six. Mum would get the kids to set the table while she got cooking. It worked every time.' – *Kay Iles*

Always get up from the dinner table feeling as if you could have eaten a little bit more.

'The fact was, we were a large family and it was a struggle to make ends meet, so there often wasn't anything left over. This made it fairly easy to follow Mum's advice! The same advice had been handed down from her mother and her grandmother, both of whom had lived through war. At various stages, basic staples were in short supply and necessities like tea, butter, sugar and flour were often rationed. By coming up with their tip, they were empowering their family to make a choice about how much they did or didn't eat, turning a negative situation into something that could be viewed with a more positive outlook.' – *Susan Belperio*

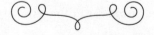

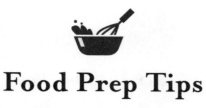

Food Prep Tips

Always prepare bread-and-butter pudding either the morning of the day it's to be cooked, or the night before. The bread needs to soak up the liquid for the best results. Also, stale bread must be used for the same reason.

'This tip came from my grandmother. I always follow her advice and so do most people I know.'
– *Irene Whennan*

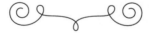

Cut onions underwater in the sink. This way, the onions release their fragrance into the water – no more crying eyes. Once peeled, simply lift out the onion peels and throw them away. Then you can slice your onions underwater and lift out onto a plate ready to use. I usually have a paper towel on the plate to pat the onions dry. It's easy and quick – no mess and no tears.

'My mother, Maureen Saxburg, started her career without any training. She started as a kitchen-hand peeling vegetables in a hospital in Sydney. One day the head cook fell ill and the staff wondered what they would do. Mother, who really was a very smart lady with lots of good-old common sense, took charge straight away and set all the cooks to work. She put another woman in charge of peeling vegetables and, when my mother saw her crying while cutting up onions, she showed her and the other cooks how to cut onions without tears, and to get on with the job. My mother was promoted to head cook, went on to complete her studies and become an A Class Cook. She worked for that hospital for 20 years. She, of course, passed her skills on to her daughter, me. And I passed them on to my girls.' – *Marilyn Featon*

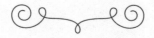

When making chips, cut them to the desired size and wrap in a tea towel or paper towel. Get the oil very hot and put in chips for 5 to 7 minutes. Then, take out and place on paper towel to drain well. Return to the hot oil until cooked. They will be the best, crispiest chips ever.

'Mum was a pretty basic cook, usually meat and three veg. I think she got this chip method from the *Sun* in Melbourne, where they had great recipes every week that people would send in and win a prize for the best.' – *Sharon Crowe*

To keep iceberg lettuce crisp, rinse under cold water after removing the core. Shake excess water away, then wrap in 2 to 3 sheets of paper towel, put in a plastic bag and place in the fridge crisper. If needed, you can refresh the lettuce a second time this way.

'This tip was handed down by my mother, who lived in a remote farming community. This meant food had to be kept as fresh as possible until the next shopping day. I always store the lettuce this way without fail, and fondly recall memories of learning to cook by observing and helping my mother in her country kitchen.' – *Janice Gaetti*

6 things you didn't know your rice cooker could make

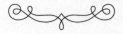

You'd be forgiven for thinking your humble rice cooker is a one-trick pony. After all, the name implies that it performs a highly specific function with no mention of anything else. Interestingly, though, the rice cooker can be used for a whole range of culinary tasks above and beyond cooking your basmati. Here are six of our favourite dishes to cook in the rice cooker.

1. Frittata
Bake a perfect frittata by simply switching to the cook setting, heat olive oil, add veggies followed by beaten eggs, cover and reset to let the cycle run through.

2. Macaroni and cheese
Super simple with minimal mess. Add all the ingredients and set to cook. Perfect mac and cheese with minimal washing up!

3. Cheesecake and banana bread
Line the rice cooker insert with baking paper. Prepare your recipe as normal, pour the batter into the lined rice cooker insert then set to cook.

4. Porridge

Wake up to perfect porridge every time! Presoak steel-cut oats overnight in the rice cooker then run the cook cycle in the morning for creamy, delicious porridge.

5. Quinoa

If you fancy jumping on the quinoa train, try cooking it in your rice cooker. It cooks at the same rate as long-grain white rice so makes the perfect substitute that doesn't require any fiddly programing changes.

6. Polenta

Create creamy polenta by adding 1 cup polenta to 3 cups stock or water and set to cook. Add cheese or butter at the end, and you're done.

A guide to pairing wine with food

When it comes to selecting wines to go with your meals, there are no absolute rules – the only expert opinion that matters is your own. That said, there are choices that definitely pair better with certain dishes. Choosing wines to go with your meals can be among the more enjoyable and relaxing stages in planning the dinner.

Where to start

Welcoming guests with flutes of crisp sparkling wine always creates a nice sense of occasion, whether your hors d'oeuvres are just some dips and crackers or a lavish selection or meat and cheeses. And if you're thinking of serving bubbles throughout an entire meal, you might be onto something. Although a soup or shellfish starter might be a sparkling's ideal partner, its bubbly assertiveness allows sparkling wine to hold its own with more robust dishes, too.

The basics

At a minimum, you want to provide refreshment – water and wines – that flatter a meal's flavours. In many cases, a good-quality, medium-bodied red wine is a great choice with meats and hearty dishes. A dry or fruity white wine goes well with lighter meals, such as fish, chicken and salads.

Provide options

A traditional roast dinner with baked vegetables – a popular
meal choice when hosting – tests the liveliness of a single wine,
so often it makes sense to offer two or more. That way, guests
can sip from whichever glass suits what they're eating.

Red hot

A red wine made substantially from pinot noir grapes is a fine
partner for the distinctive taste of dark meat, and the black
cherry-like character of many pinot noirs will evoke the rich
berry sauces popular throughout the cooler months of the year.
With a broad range of flavours in your meals, you may want to
introduce maturity and complexity in your wines. Try either the
sun-baked earthiness of a shiraz or a rioja, or the hint of mellow
age found in wines older than four or five years.

The white note

A well-crafted white wine can be a star of a dinner table,
especially if it picks up on the citrus tones that are often present
in sauces and garnishes of meals. Rich, concentrated white
wines, such as a viognier or a chardonnay, with higher alcohol
and a wisp of butterscotch sweetness, can enhance white meat.
If the white is elegant and floral enough, it can be the perfect
chaser for more herbal dishes, too.

Set a budget

With very little legwork, you can find wines like these in every
price range, so once you've decided on your menu and before
you commit to certain wines, sample a few options.

How to combat wine stains

When it comes to dinner-party disasters, top of the list is usually a red wine spill on cream-coloured carpet. Mothers know how to get these stubborn stains out of clothing and carpets, and now you will too.

Method 1 – Clothing: First, blot up as much of the stain as possible using paper towel or an old towel. Then cover the stained area generously with soda water, which will help break up the stain. Wash clothing as normal.

Method 2 – Carpets: After blotting up the stain with paper towel, sprinkle bicarb soda over the stain and leave to absorb any remaining liquid. Once dry, vacuum over the area. If any faint stain lingers, dab at area with a cloth dampened with white vinegar.

Here's a trick for when you need to clean up large quantities of spilled liquids, such as beer or soft drink, from carpet. Grab an old towel, place it over the spill still-folded and walk on it. The repeated pressure from your feet aids the blotting action of the towel and lifts the spill in no time. Once the spill is removed, wash area with cold water and a little dish liquid and repeat the stepping action to dry.

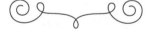

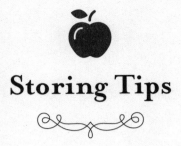

Storing Tips

5 ways to make your groceries last longer

Back in the days of war when people had to live off rations and little else, mothers were skilled at making things last. Cut back on how much you're throwing out by storing your groceries correctly and effectively, from the moment you return from the shops. We've all cleaned out the fridge and realised just how much food we've wasted through improper storage. Here are five tips to prevent this and make your groceries last longer.

1. Bread

Is your bread constantly going mouldy? It's probably because you're storing it somewhere damp. Bread is best kept in a bread bin or similar cool-dry place. To keep it much longer, freeze it.

2. Celery

We've all bought a bunch of celery only to find it soggy and wilted 25 hours later. The best way to store celery is actually to wrap the whole thing, top to bottom, in foil! Wrap and pop it in the fridge for longer-lasting crunchy fronds.

3. Berries

Have you been removing your strawberries from the punnet? Don't! Berry punnets are designed to prevent ethylene gas (which causes fruit to ripen and eventually rot) from becoming trapped. Transferring your berries to an airtight container will actually make them spoil faster, as the gas has nowhere to go.

4. Apples

You can keep apples in the fridge or on the benchtop but, make sure you inspect them regularly. One mouldy apple can spoil the whole bowl/crisper as it will release huge amounts of ethylene gas. If you notice an apple on the turn, bin it immediately!

5. Tomato paste

It's frustrating having to open a whole tin of tomato paste when all you require is a tablespoon or two. Make the rest last longer by spooning it into an ice cube tray and freezing. That way, you can pop out a cube whenever you need a small amount.

How to keep an avocado for up to six months

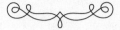

Australians have a love affair with avocados. When prices are low and supply is plentiful, stock up on your favourite food and store it in the freezer. Yes – as it turns out, you can freeze avocados for up to six months following these four steps.

1. Wash the ripe avocado, skin on. Cut in half, peel and remove pit.

2. Wrap each half in foil or plastic wrap then place them in a zip-lock bag labelled with the date (so you'll know how long they've been in the freezer).

3. If you'd rather pureed avocado, mash with a bit of lemon juice, lime juice or white vinegar, then place in the freezer in a zip-lock bag or airtight container labelled with the date.

4. To thaw; move avocado to fridge about 12 to 24 hours before use; leave at room temperature for an hour; or put in a bowl and run cold water over the bag or container.

As great as this technique is for avid avocado eaters, it comes with a word of warning: thawed avocado won't be as firm as fresh. However, for those of us who love a bit of guacamole or smashed-avo on toast, this money-saving trick is a godsend.

Freezer know-how

You can freeze all manner of fruit, vegetables and herbs when in season, to enjoy later on when they're unavailable in the shops.

Freezing vegetables

As a general rule, most sturdy vegetables, such as carrots, broccoli, peas, corn, asparagus, capsicum, green beans, potatoes, sweet potato and mushrooms, can be frozen. Blanch or steam first so they are tender crisp, then store in zip-lock bags labelled with the date. Soft, watery veggies like lettuces and tomatoes are not suitable.

Freezing fruit

To minimise browning, use only ripe, unblemished fruit and dip in a mixture of water and lemon juice before freezing. Apples, stone fruit, such as peaches and mangoes, and berries can all be frozen. Slice larger fruits or arrange whole berries on baking trays to freeze, then place in zip-lock bags labelled with the date.

Freezing herbs

There's nothing more wasteful than buying a bunch of herbs for a single meal, then leaving them to wilt in the fridge. You can freeze whole sprigs of herbs in zip-lock bags (wash thoroughly first). Or, chop herbs and pack into ice-cube trays, cover with a little water and freeze. Once frozen, turn out into a zip-lock bag and label with the date.

Cooking Tips

6 tips for cooking the perfect steak

Why is it that we can rarely cook a steak at home that's as delicious as a steak from a restaurant? It seems that the chefs at the local steakhouse are wise to a few insider tips that we can now share with you. Get your tongs ready ...

1. Ensure the meat is at room temperature

How many times have we broken this rule? Letting your meat come to room temperature before it hits the grill or BBQ is important, as it ensures your steak cooks more evenly all the way through.

2. Get your grill super hot

If you don't, you won't get that nice charred outer edge on your steak that helps to hold in moisture. But don't leave the steak on the super heat for too long – just enough to sear the meat. Then turn down the heat a little to allow it to cook through.

3. Season to perfection

While your BBQ heats up, be sure to season both sides of your steak with salt and pepper. Many home cooks season only one side, or forget to season at all.

4. Test for doneness with your fingers

Many of us are guilty of poking a steak with a fork to see whether it's cooked. But this just means the steak starts to lose moisture. Instead, feel the steak with your hand – if it's soft, it's rare, and if it's firm to touch, it's well done.

5. Avoid too much turning or pressing

A steak only needs to be cooked on each side, not continually turned. Too much flipping is another way a steak loses moisture, and we want that to stay inside. Same goes with pressing down on the steak – that sizzle you hear is moisture escaping from the meat. It's a no no.

6. Give your steak a rest

After all that cooking, your steak needs a few minutes to rest before serving. Don't just pop it on somebody's plate straight from the BBQ. About 10 minutes should do it. Then season the steak again before plating up.

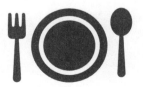

Baking Tips

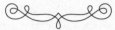

When making pastry for an apple tart or slice, add a tablespoon of custard powder to the flour.

'No idea who I got this one from. It just makes the pastry and apple taste special.' – *Karen Murdock*

When making a cake, don't rinse out the bowl with hot water – always use cold water. Hot water cooks the cake mix to the side of the bowl, and it's harder to wash up the bowl than if you rinse with cold water first.

'My grandma and I were making cupcakes in her big old kitchen when she told me about this little cleaning tip.' – *Janette Newman*

Make sponge cakes with custard powder and cornflower, and they will always be light and fluffy.

'My mother-in-law taught me to cook. I used to love to watch her cooking – she was a very patient and talented lady. She also taught me how to sew. I miss her very much.' – *Carolyn Southurst*

Save your used butter paper to line your square cake tin.

'Although I don't remember cooking with my mother, I must have learnt this from her.'
– *Benita Buchanan*

When cutting scones from scone dough, always use an open-top cutter because the scones won't rise otherwise.

'This came from my mother, who was born in Australia in 1913. She worked and raised five children on cattle properties in the bush, while supporting her husband. She won many an award for her scones. Love and miss my mum every day.'
– *Nerida Irwin*

What to do when you're short an ingredient or two

It's happened to us all: we've gathered together everything to bake a cake or muffins only to discover there's only one egg and no self-raising flour.

Fear not! Here's a handy list of substitutes and make-dos to save a mad dash to the shops.

And while we're at it, baking soda is the same thing as bicarbonate of soda, but both are *different* from baking powder!

Missing ingredient	Magic make-do
Arrowroot	Use cornflour or tapioca starch
Baking powder	To replace 1 teaspoon, add 1/4 teaspoon bicarbonate of soda to 1/2 teaspoon cream of tartar
Buttermilk	Add 1 tablespoon lemon juice to 1 cup skim milk, or use 1 cup yogurt (for a thicker mixture)
Cooking chocolate	For 30 g, add 4 tablespoons cocoa powder and 1 teaspoon caster sugar to 1 tablespoon butter or oil
Cream cheese	Use cottage cheese or natural yogurt strained overnight
Crème fraiche	Use sour cream or natural yogurt
Egg	For one egg, add 1 tablespoon chia seeds to 3 tablespoons water
Golden syrup	For 1/2 cup, use a scant 1/2 cup honey topped up with molasses
Self-raising flour	Add 2 teaspoons baking powder to 1 cup plain flour

Cake decorating 101

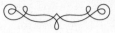

When decorating your baked goods, there are many tips and tricks to help you create a masterpiece. But before you get to the fun part, ensure your cakes are looking professional rather than disastrous with these basics.

DECORATING TOOLS

1. Sturdy serrated knife (to ensure clean cuts)
2. Large and small offset spatulas (to make precise icing easy)
3. Teaspoon and table knife (in place of more specialised tools)
4. Pastry bags (to make icing and create patterns or shapes)
5. Rubber spatula (to stir batter)
6. Bamboo skewers (to stabilise cake layers – not always required)

DECORATING TIPS

Buttering up

Remove the butter for both your cake and icing from the fridge about an hour before you start cooking, to allow it to be room temperature. This will ensure your butter is soft enough to beat and create a light, fluffy texture.

Prepping perfection

Make the cake at least one day before you intend to cut it into shapes. This will make cutting easier. You can store cakes, before icing them, in an airtight container for up to two days.

Colouring icing

Adding colour to your icing comes in two forms – gel or paste.
At this step, one of the most important things to remember is
that a little goes a long way. Swirl a toothpick into the colouring
and mix well into your icing. Add the colour little by little until
you have your desired hue. There's also liquid food colouring,
which is commonly found in supermarkets, but it only comes
in limited colours, such as red, blue, yellow and green. To use,
stir drops of food colouring into the icing (mix and match the
primary colours to get creative hues!) until you achieve your
desired colour.

Flavouring icing

For a little something extra, you can add flavour to your icing
to complement the flavour of the cake. Choose from flavourings
and extracts (such as vanilla, almond, rum or maple), liqueurs
(such as raspberry, hazelnut or coffee) and different citrus zests
to add standout flavours before decorating your cake.

Using a coupler

The plastic coupler is a nifty little tool that allows you to use
different decorating tips while piping from one bag.
To change decorating tips, unscrew the coupler ring,
replace the decorating tip and replace the ring. Voila.

Filling a pastry bag

First, you need to place the bag, tip down, in a tall glass and cuff
the bag around the rim. Insert icing with a spatula, scraping
against the side of the bag to release the icing. Be sure not to

fill the bag more than halfway. Unfold the cuff. Gather the top edges together with one hand and, with the other hand, drag the thumb and index finger downwards, letting out air and forcing the icing into the bag and decorating tip. Twist the top of the bag to close and to maintain pressure.

Creating the perfect base

To ensure your icing experience is seamless and doesn't get too messy, it's important that every icing job begins with a smooth layer of base icing.

1. Place the chilled cake on a cardboard cake round or plate, and transfer it to a rotating cake stand. Smooth on a base layer of slightly chilled buttercream with a straight icing spatula to seal the cake crumbs. Chill the cake until icing has hardened; this should take about 15 minutes.

2. Next, you'll want to coat the sides of the cake with 5–6 mm of buttercream. Hold the icing spatula parallel to the sides of the cake, with the blade slightly angled towards you. Apply pressure against the sides of the cake with the spatula and use your other hand to rotate the cake stand, smoothing the sides.

3. Spread excess icing from the sides onto the top of the cake and add more to coat. Position the spatula almost flat, halfway across the top of the cake. Apply pressure as you rotate the cake stand, smoothing the top. Chill until the icing has hardened, about 15 minutes, before decorating.

Basic buttercream

125 g unsalted butter, softened

1½ cups icing sugar, sifted

1 teaspoon vanilla extract

1 tablespoon milk

Using a wooden spoon or electric mixer, beat the butter until pale and creamy. Slowly spoon in the icing sugar, beating well between each addition. Add vanilla and a little milk, just enough to make mixture spreadable.

This buttercream is a great base icing for adding colours and other flavours. To make a chocolate buttercream, for example, add 25–30 g melted cooking chocolate to the mixture.

Foolproof icing glaze

1½ cups icing sugar

2–3 tablespoons water

1 teaspoon vanilla extract

Sift the icing sugar into a mixing bowl. Slowly add water and vanilla, a teaspoon at a time, until the mixture reaches a smooth consistency.

To make a tangy citrus glaze, omit the vanilla extract and replace water with freshly squeezed lime or lemon juice.

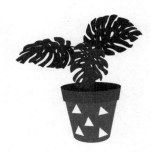

Around the house

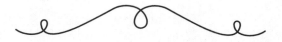

'I've been influenced by women all my life; not that men, like my dad, didn't offer inspiration, but it was and remains ladies who direct my day-to-day life. As a child, and I mean from two to three when I started to talk, my nana taught me how to talk to plants (an early guidance on my career). My dear mother, who made stunning sponges and cupcakes for school fetes but never ate one (something I failed to learn), was strong. She washed, ironed and vacuumed, spoke eloquently, respected others, always punched well above her 'weight' and got involved in community – all of which has become my life's mantra to this day. My wife of nearly 50 years has kept me focused, my daughter offers endless encouragement and my granddaughter gives me the energy to try and achieve.'

— *Graham Ross, Australian horticulturalist, author and television presenter*

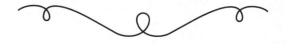

Cleaning Tips

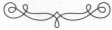

When cleaning the house, carry a small basket with you from room to room – if you find something where it shouldn't be, put it in the basket and replace it in its correct spot when you enter that room. Makes it easy to keep your home looking tidy at least – without having stray shoes and toys lying about, or bathroom and laundry items sitting in the kitchen.

'Mum had a good rule when we were kids – "Don't put it down, put it away." – but we all know how easy it is to get side-tracked from tasks. Sadly, Mum is in a nursing home these days with dementia, but her common sense and practical advice still help to keep us on track.' – *Maureen Clifford*

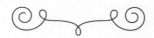

Dancing to music while wearing socks on your feet helps to clean timber and tiled floors.

'When living and sharing with others, it's always important to be considerate. Just part of life's skills!'
– *Margaret Besomo*

Your clothes are only as clean as the last rinsing water used. Floors are only as clean as the utensil (broom, mop or vacuum cleaner) you use to clean it with. Always dust with a clean duster. When washing or painting a wall, do the outsides edges first and the centre will be almost done.

These rules came down the generations from mums, except for the one about the centre. My dad used to say, "Do things from the outside first and the centre will take care of itself."' – *Lily Ayling*

Use vinegar daily for just about everything –
cleaning, disinfecting and health. My personal
favourite is to use it in the washing machine
instead of fabric softener. That one I told my
mum about.

'Mum taught me about vinegar and I have passed it
on to my children.' – *Margret McPharlin*

Make sure you tidy up before you go to bed.
If anything should happen to you during the
night, you don't want people to remember that
you didn't keep a good house.

'My mother was of Irish descent and had some really
funny sayings like, "If I catch you up doing that
again, I will pay you." We would run away laughing,
saying, "How much will you pay us, Mum?" I smile
each time I think of that.' – *Mary. T. Jones*

Always ensure your sink is clear of dirty dishes and the beds are made.

'This tip, or rather instruction, came from my mum when I was a child. I was frequently "encouraged" to make my bed before leaving for school. The areas mentioned are, of course, highly visible and really do stand out if not done. Mum always finished the instruction with the words, "If this is done, you can get away with anything else."' – *Sally Mayocchi*

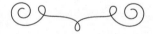

Bicarbonate of soda tips

Always keep a box of bicarbonate of soda in the pantry as it has many uses. It's a great odour remover for furniture, mattresses or in the car. Sprinkle dry bicarb over the offending area, allow it to sit for a while and then vacuum off. You can also use it in the bath for irritated and itchy skin.

'Becoming a first-time mum has it challenges. When Bubs was sick in the night on the cot mattress, Mum gave me this tip and it worked wonders to remove the odour – no more bad smells!' – *Jo Scott*

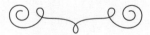

Bring bicarb soda with you when you shower and give it a clean while you're in it. A few minutes regularly will save you from having to do a big clean later.

'I began doing this when I had five children under 10, as it's a real time-saver.' – *Carol Huber*

After you clean your oven, cover the oven floor with bicarb and leave it there. It collects the grease when you cook next time. Then to clean, you just sprinkle vinegar over, let it sit for a few minutes and scrape it up. Wipe out with a hot cloth. This one works for cleaning sinks or saucepans, too.

'From my family.' – *Rod Hyde*

10 brilliant ways to clean with coconut oil

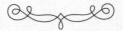

While you may have been aware that coconut oil is a miracle in the kitchen and a godsend in the beauty department, you might not have known that it's also pretty handy as a cleaning agent! We've rounded up our 10 favourite ways to use this nifty oil around the home.

1. Polish timber
Give tired old timber furniture a quick refresh with a dollop of coconut oil.

2. Season a frypan
Season and restore your frypan by lightly coating with some coconut oil. You'll need to heat the pan to melt the oil, then leave to cool.

3. Condition leather
Leather lounge looking less than lustrous? A soft cloth and a dollop of coconut oil will help to restore shine.

4. Remove sticky labels
Mix coconut oil, bicarb soda and lemon juice to remove sticky label leftovers from bottles, plastic and other hard surfaces.

5. Condition wooden kitchen implements

Hydrate your chopping board, salad bowl or wood spoons by gently applying a generous dollop of coconut oil and buffing in with a soft cloth.

6. Say 'sayonara' to rust

Apply coconut oil to tarnished silverware or rusty scissors to remove rust and restore shine. Let sit for 30 minutes then rinse well.

7. Make your own hand cream

Coconut oil mixed with a few drops of your favourite essential oil makes for the perfect nourishing hand cream. Warm the oil until just melting, add essential oil then leave to cool before use.

8. Remove crayon marks

Grandkids decided to decorate your kitchen wall or bench with their crayons? Remove the offending stains with a few dabs of coconut oil and a sponge.

9. Wax your car

If you want to avoid harsh chemical-laden car products, try coconut oil for your interior, dash, steering wheel and exterior.

10. Make homemade baby wipes

Steer clear of chemicals by creating a baby-wipe solution out of coconut oil, chamomile, hot water and a splash of baby shampoo. To use, simply dip a make-up remover pad into the mixture.

Never go anywhere empty handed; use your head to save your feet when moving from one room to another, or from the house to the yard.

'Mum had eight children and also brought up one grandchild; as we grew older, she worked part-time. She lived by and imparted the above tip. Today I am compiling her eulogy and this was one thing that came to mind.' – *Sharyn Copley*

Mum always told me to stand the broom up, it saves the bristles from curling.

'Because they saw me standing the broom up the wrong way.' – *Chris Smith*

The Way Mum Does It

To easily remove the smells that bleach, onion and garlic leave on your hands, place your hands under cool water and rub all over with a stainless-steel spoon. The odour will completely disappear.

'My grandma led a reasonably frugal country life, where cleaning and cooking were part of daily life. Being able to use gloves or scented soaps were luxuries. She told me not to ask how this worked, just be happy you know it does.' – *Marlene Cochrane*

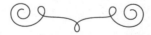

5 tips to get rid of kitchen odours

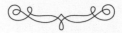

Some kitchen aromas are rather lovely – the smell of Grandma's famous lamb roast wafting from the oven or the sweet scent of Mum's freshly baked apple pie. Then there are the other smells – which can be a bit nasty – that can be hard to get rid of. Follow our tips to get your kitchen smelling great again.

1. Keep your fridge clean

Ensure your refrigerator is regularly cleaned. Take everything out and make your own cleaning spray, by mixing 3 tablespoons bicarb soda into a spray bottle of water. Spray the inside of the fridge, including the shelves, and wipe it clean with a sponge. To keep your fridge fresh, pop a cup of bicarb inside to absorb some of that 'fridge smell', replacing it every three months.

2. Clean your drains

Drains and garbage disposals can trap bad smells inside. Keep them clear by pouring 3 tablespoons bicarb soda down the drain every month. Leave it for 10 minutes then pour in 1/2 cup white vinegar. It will fizz up and clear out any stuck-on grime. Rinse with hot water. If you have a garbage disposal, send down a cup of warm water and a chopped-up lemon once a week to combat any odours trapped inside.

3. Freshen up your bin

Keep the garbage bin and recycling bin in the kitchen clean by swishing them with either vinegar and water, or a germ-killing disinfectant. If you notice a spill in the bin, take it outside and rinse well with water before leaving it to dry in the sun.

4. Make ovens and stovetops shine

Grease and food spills on your stovetop or in your oven can become truly smelly areas. If your stovetop needs a scrub, try using half vinegar and half water to cut through grease and grime. For an alternative to the fume-filled oven cleaners, make your own with baking soda mixed with water to make a paste. Wipe onto the oven, allow to dry and then use a clean damp cloth to wipe it off again.

5. Keep sponges fresh

Your sponge is a breeding ground for bacteria and therefore odours, so it's important to keep sponges in good shape. Germs in the sponge can make your family ill, so it's not just the smell that's the issue. Choose cellulose sponges and remember to pop them in the dishwasher every few days to keep clean. Another trick is to wet a sponge, squeeze out the excess water, and then microwave it on high for 2 minutes to remove bacteria.

Always use the right tool for the job, keep it sharp (if necessary) and always clean your tools before putting them away.

'I used to love playing in the garage when Dad was tinkering with things. As he died young, those memories became more precious and his advice has always stood me in good stead.' – *Joy Dixon*

Cooking salt rubbed into stained tea or coffee cups removes the stain.

'This came from my father's mother, who kept an immaculately clean home.' – *Robyn Phillips*

To clean oven racks, soak them in water with washing soda – overnight is best. The grime will then fall off with a cloth.

'My mother told me this tip and it works so well. My mother was a "girl who can do anything" type of person who lived and fought in WWII. She always said, "We don't have to wait around for a man to do anything."' – *E.J. Russell*

To clean a burnt saucepan, fill the saucepan halfway, bring to the boil and add vinegar. Remove the saucepan from the heat and add bicarb soda. Let mixture stand overnight. Empty the saucepan and scour as normal.

'My nan taught me to cook when I was 10. I had many a disaster so she also taught me how to clean the saucepan.' – *Kay Feain*

3 tips to clean stains from baking trays

It may be one of your least-favourite jobs but cleaning your baking trays is unfortunately a necessity. Burnt food, grease and grime can accumulate quickly on this kitchen workhorse, especially if you're leaving it awhile between scrubbings. Sadly, a dishwasher just can't apply the same kind of focused pressure that manual scrubbing can. Fortunately, you can return your trays to their former glory with a little bit of elbow grease and some cleaning know-how. Here are our top three tips for removing tough stains.

1. **If you're dealing with a greasy tray or burnt and blackened** food, ensure you remove any big clumps from the tray with paper towel. You don't need to scrub, just remove as much grease or loose soot as possible.

2. **For a greasy tray,** fill your kitchen sink with piping hot water and add a good squirt of a concentrated dishwashing liquid. Pop the tray in and soak for a couple of hours or even overnight. Once the grease has softened, use a soft sponge or cloth (for a non-stick tray) or a more robust sponge or scourer (for a regular tray) to remove remaining grease and oil. Once you've done the hard yards, pop into the dishwasher to remove any last traces of residue.

3. For a charred tray, the best technique uses baking soda and hot water. Boil your kettle then fill the sink with the hot water. Add a cup of baking soda and wait for the bubbles to subside. Pop your tray into the sink and leave for an hour or longer. Once the crusts have softened, wipe away with a dishcloth or sponge, then pop into the dishwasher for a sparkling clean tray.

Time-saving tray tips

To minimise the amount of grease and residue that build up on your baking trays, season them with coconut or olive oil before use. The greasy mess will then just wash away with hot water, saving you the trouble of scrubbing each time.

Also, don't forget to line your trays with baking paper – it's not just for cakes! A dab or two of oil on the tray will keep the paper in place nicely.

Pour white vinegar into the toilet cistern before going to bed. When you flush it in the morning, you will be amazed!

'This tip was passed to me by my mother.'
– *Marg Rouse*

Mix equal parts of white vinegar with water to clean your computer screen, reading glasses and other glass. Buff with a microfibre cloth to finish. A spray bottle is the best thing to store and use when needed.

'My lovely mother gave me this useful tip one day when she saw how smeary my computer screen was. She found a small spray bottle then and there, and mixed the solution up. In a minute I had a beautiful clean, shiny screen.' – *Mary Hart*

A mixture of eucalyptus oil and shampoo will remove greasy marks.

'From my grandma.' – *Lynn Poupart*

To clean a microwave, cut a lemon in half, microwave for 40 seconds, remove, then wipe the inside of the microwave with a damp cloth. Too easy.

'From my mum, who has passed on.' – *Joye Rieger*

To remove pet hair from clothes or furniture, wear a pair of kitchen rubber gloves and just brush it away with your hands. Using your hands like a brush, the hairs just roll together for easy removal. – *Elaine Napier*

The easiest way to clean your mattress

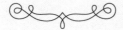

You change your sheets regularly but what about your poor-old mattress? Not only does your mattress do all the hard work, supporting through your nights of slumber, it can also benefit from a deep clean. Mattresses are prime spots for dust build-up, largely because we don't think to clean them very often. Cleaning your mattress with the mixture below helps to lift away dirt and dust, while removing excess moisture and giving it a general refreshing.

People with allergies, such as asthma and hay fever, often find that a mattress spring-clean does wonders for their airways. Although, anyone can benefit from a bedding refresh! Here's how to do it.

What you'll need:
- 500 g box bicarbonate of soda
- Essential oil(s) of your choice (such as lavender, chamomile and ylang ylang)
- Vacuum cleaner (with an upholstery nozzle, if you have one)

How to:

1. Before you start, it's a good idea to turn and rotate your mattress, especially if you haven't done so in a while. You should try to do this every six months but many of us forget.

2. Open your box of bicarb soda and add 10–20 drops of your chosen essential oil, or blend of oils. Go for something soothing and calming. You could also add tea tree and/or eucalyptus oil for their anti-bacterial properties.

3. Liberally sprinkle the bicarb soda over your mattress. Don't be shy! Once you've emptied the box, start rubbing the mixture into the mattress. This ensures that it reaches into all the cracks and crevices.

4. After 1–2 hours, start vacuuming up the residue. Use your upholstery nozzle or brush attachment and work slowly to ensure you hoover up all the bicarb mixture.

Sponge secrets

Microfibre dish sponges and cloths are a terrific alternative to the old throwaway sponge or Chux. These clean crockery gently and some have built-in scourers for tougher debris. Just throw them in the washing machine every couple of days and reuse them. No more disgusting disintegrating sponges!

Once your sponge is on its last cleaning legs, you still don't need to throw it away. After cleaning in the microwave (blast on 'high' for 30–60 seconds) or washing machine, try one of these ideas:

1. Line the bottom of houseplant pots to help retain moisture in the potting mix.

2. Use as the substrate for a miniature garden – lay on a small plate or soap dish, moisten with water, sprinkle your seeds on top, cover with an upside down glass bowl then watch your sprouts grow.

3. Cut an old foam sponge into shapes (square, circle, triangle, etc.) and use as paint sponges.

4. Got a mouse problem? Try soaking scraps of old sponge in peppermint oil and stuffing these into mouse holes. The strong-smelling peppermint is thought to confuse the mice into staying away.

When using the clothes dryer, soak a Chux in fabric softener then wring it out. Put the Chux in the dryer with the clothes and your clothes will come out soft and smelling lovely. It also reduces static.

'A girlfriend who was doing it tough years ago shared this tip with me. I couldn't believe it worked so well and it saved a lot of fabric softener as well.'
– *Eileen Tennant*

When washing curtains, don't hang them on the line to dry and then iron them. Hang them back up while still damp and they won't have any creases in them.

'My mother, who has passed, gave me this fabulous tip when I was about to wash some curtains one day. It works and is a time-saver.' – *Brenda Smith*

8 washing tips to make your whites whiter and your colours brighter

Here we have eight Mum-approved tips for washing. Taking the time to wash your clothes carefully means they'll look their best and last much longer.

1. Act fast to remove stains from fabric. The longer you leave it, the harder it is to remove.

2. Remove spilled liquids on fabric by blotting with a white cloth or paper towel. Start on the outside of the stain and work your way in to the centre, so the stain doesn't spread.

3. Help to remove an oily stain by sprinkling it with cornflour. Leave for 15 minutes before scraping it off and laundering as usual.

4. Use fresh lemon to help whiten your napkins, linen placemats or even sports socks. On the stovetop, fill a large pot with water and add some sliced lemon. Bring water to the boil then turn off the heat. Add your whites and soak for an hour before washing as normal.

5. Many stains benefit from a bit of bicarb. Make a paste of 3 tablespoons bicarb soda and 3 tablespoons water. Place the paste over the affected area and leave to sit for 15 minutes before washing.

6. Clean white tablecloths by adding 1/4 cup white vinegar to your rinse cycle. White vinegar cuts through grease and can help to remove stubborn stains such as red wine or tomato sauce.

7. Before washing your clothes, close all zippers, clasps, hooks and snaps to prevent them snagging on other items. However, leave buttons undone, it's better for your clothes.

8. Protect the fabric on fade-prone clothes, such as dark trousers or jeans, by washing them inside out.

For best results in the wash, use eucalyptus oil and bicarbonate of soda.

'This tip was passed down from Nanna.'
– *John Langham*

Forget about all the supermarket stain removers for clothes; just rub a squirt of dishwashing liquid on the stain and pop in the wash. Works every time.

'A good friend passed this tip on to me after I was complaining about ruining my new shirt, which had a huge stain from spaghetti bolognaise sauce. It came out brilliantly. So that's all I use now. Any dishwashing liquid will do, but I prefer Palmolive.'
– *Jen Slater*

Clean oily stains on your garments made of any fabric (silk, crepe, cotton) by generously covering the stain with baby powder. Next, cover the powdered stain with a handkerchief and iron over the handkerchief, checking it once or twice. Once the oil is absorbed, take off the handkerchief and use it to rub the remaining baby powder gently. Finished!

'My mother first gave me this tip when I was a teenager. I'd come home from a party and found an oily stain on my gown. My late mum had always been well informed about everything. I love her!'
— *Setyowati Soepadnomo*

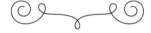

To clean the dirty mark from inside a shirt collar, first wet, rub with washing soap (Sunlite, in those days) and sprinkle with sugar. Leave for an hour or so and wash off.

'This was something my mother did. My father worked in a foundry when we were small and his shirt collars always had a ring of dirt along the inside after a day's work. Worked a treat and when I need to, I still do it. My mum passed away 14 years ago at the age of 88.' – *Shirley Duncan*

Fold your sheets top to bottom and peg to the line, not folded in half over the line. It is easier for one person to get off.

'My grandmother came to stay and showed me this trick. I have done this from when I got married to now.' – *Barbara Whitfield*

Before putting dirty towels in the wash, my mum would use them (dry or still slightly damp) for wiping ceramic tiles, taps and surfaces, and for dusting furniture and surfaces. This way they get an efficient and timesaving double use before washing.

'I immigrated to Australia from Canada with my Australian husband. At that time, the hardest day in my life was telling my parents that we would be going to live on the other side of the world, taking their beloved grandchildren with us. We would try and visit each other as often as possible but, as you can imagine, the cost of airfares for two adults and two children was pretty steep. On one of our visits to Canada, I insisted on doing the weekly clean for my mum so she could spend the time with her grandchildren, and she gave me the above tip. I've used it ever since. It really is a time-saver and is very efficient.' – *Roslyn McLaren*

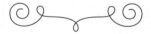

When pegging out blouses, T-shirts and so on, put the peg in the armpit. You won't see the peg mark under the arm.

'My mother-in-law gave me this tip many years ago. I've now passed it on to my daughter.'
– *Rosalind Higginson*

Hang your suede or corduroy skirts and jackets in the bathroom while you shower or bathe. It will freshen them up and take out any creases.

'Passed on to me by my grandmother, who had been a seamstress.' – *Elizabeth Newington*

Always iron shirts in this order: yoke, collar, cuffs, sleeves and then side, back and side. For handkerchiefs, iron all four edges first, then the middle, then top to bottom, bottom to top, left to right and right to left.

'My mum was old school. I had three brothers and I remember getting really cranky about ironing their shirts. Mum was a ladies' maid for a while and learnt her laundry skills from the housekeeper. She actually loved ironing and was doing ironing for people when she was in her eighties, right up until three months before she died. And she did it for people she loved. I'm afraid I'm not so altruistic, although I still iron things this way. I can hear her instructions in my head as if it were yesterday.' – *Lyn Whiteway*

When the bottom of your iron has suffered because you've ironed something on too hot a temperature – spray it with oven cleaner. Works like a charm.

'My good friend Deb Flood told me this tip, and it really works.' – *Robyn Hayes*

Place matching sheets and one pillowcase inside the other pillowcase to keep sets together for easy storage and practical use. Also, roll towels up in the linen press for easy matching and storage. It takes up less space to roll towels and bath mats. And it looks neat and tidy, too.

'My daughter Bernadette, now 36, worked in Target when she was in the latter stages of high school and during her university studies. She worked in the manchester department. My friends often commented what a pleasure it was to shop there and find what they were looking for. Bernadette passed these tips on to me 15 years ago and I've found them really useful. These daughter-to-mother tips are much appreciated and valued as we pass them on to family and friends.' – *Marie Hills*

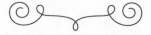

When stitching bottoms onto a garment, double the thread; this strengthens the attachment and halves the time and effort. Also, when placing cut flowers in a vase, remove all leaves from the stem area, which will be immersed in water; this prolongs the life of the flowers.

'Believe it or not, my daughter gave me these hints. Knowledge can flow both ways.' – *Maureen Calaby*

The inside of a banana peel will polish brown shoes to perfection.

'My Northern Irish great granny had her very first banana at the age of 89. She dropped the peel on her late husband's shoes (which were kept by the front door to deter intruders). When she bent to pick up the peel, she farted and was upset and embarrassed. She tried to pretend it was the noise of the peel rubbing on the shoe. To her amazement, it polished the part of the shoe she'd wiped so she did both of them.' – *Valerie O'Doherty*

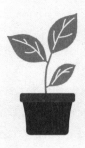

Gardening Tips

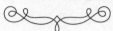

8 uses for Epsom salts in the garden

Comprised of hydrated magnesium sulphate, a naturally occurring mineral, Epsom salts are a good old-fashioned home remedy to give your garden an extra boost. Both cost effective and gentle on your greenery, here are eight uses for Epsom salts in your garden.

Note: It's always advisable to do a soil test in your garden before applying any nutrients to the soil.

1. Improve seed germination
Give your garden a boost, right from the start! Magnesium helps seed germination and strengthens cell walls. Incorporate 1 cup Epsom salts per 100 square feet of soil, or mix 1 or 2 tablespoons into the soil at the bottom of each hole before dropping in seeds.

2. Help nutrient absorption

Commercial fertilisers often add magnesium to help roots absorb nutrients, so go straight to the source. Add Epsom salts to the soil to improve absorption naturally.

3. Turn yellow foliage green

Yellowing leaves are often caused by a magnesium deficiency, as magnesium is an essential component in the production of chlorophyll. Try sprinkling 1 tablespoon Epsom salts around the soil of your plants once a month. You could also mix 1 tablespoon Epsom salts into 3 litres water and spray directly on leaves.

4. Prevent leaf curling

Leaf curling may also be caused by a lack of magnesium so sprinkle Epsom salts onto the soil around the base of the plant, or spray with the above mixture of Epsom salts and water.

5. Weed killer

This natural weed killer works a treat. In a large spray bottle, mix 2 cups Epsom salts with 4 litres vinegar and 4 tablespoons dishwashing liquid.

6. Beautiful roses

It seems the secret to beautiful roses might just be Epsom salts.
Not only do they help roses produce larger blossoms in greater
numbers, the salt makes their colour richer, foliage darker and
plants stronger. When planting, soak roots in 1/2 cup Epsom
salts diluted in 3 litres water. Also sprinkle Epsom salts in
the hole prior to planting. Once per month during growing,
sprinkle 1 tablespoon Epsom salts per foot of plant height
around the base of plant.

7. Tasty tomatoes

Tomatoes are prone to magnesium deficiency later in the
growing season. Regular applications of Epsom salts will result
in more blooms, less blossom rot and sweeter, tastier and more
bountiful tomatoes. When planting, add 1 tablespoon Epsom
salts per hole before planting seeds or transplanting. Then,
mix 1 tablespoon in 3 litres water and spray plants with solution
every two weeks.

8. Plentiful capsicums and chillies

Like tomatoes, capsicums are traditionally magnesium deficient
too, so follow the above tomato recommendations for greater
yields and stronger capsicums.

Save all your eggshells and mix them with potting mix to add calcium to the garden.

'My mother was a keen gardener and grew many beautiful plants in her cottage garden.' – *Kay Tregaskis*

Dip all your cuttings in honey and you will get a much better strike rate.

'Mum was a very keen gardener. On the farm she had a huge vegetable garden, orchard and a beautiful flower garden. I would often be woken up at first light to the sound of the shovel. She wore many shovels out, but kept us all fed with beautiful fresh fruit and vegetables.' – *Mary McEnallay*

Plant mint near the back door to keep flies away. In the old days there was no fly-screen, so all manner of insects could access the house.

'Mum grew up on a farm and many a lesson in life came from her upbringing. She grew the most fabulous vegetables, considering we grew up in North Queensland where the climate was against any vegetables surviving. But Mum had a way with herbs that deterred insects feeding on her garden.'
– *Beverley Mors*

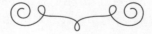

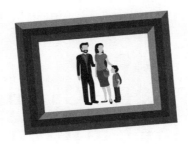

Family and relationships

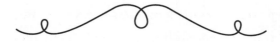

'Advice my mother gave to me: "Always treat others as you would like them to treat you."'

— Ita Buttrose, AO OBE, Australian media icon and businesswoman

Tips for Caring
for Children

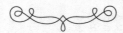

Children are given to us for a short time to love
unconditionally, to shape into caring, loving,
sensitive and responsible adults. They need
boundaries for which they will one day thank us.

'This advice was given to me by my maternal
grandmother, herself a mother to 15 children.
My own mother followed this, as I did with
my own two sons.' – *Lyn Jacklin*

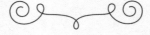

No matter how you feel after bringing your baby home, make sure you get changed out of your PJs every day. It will make you feel like you can cope with anything.

'Passed on to me by my mother, when she saw how exhausted and sore I was following a C-section.'
– *Jo Boyes*

Don't think that because the kids have left home they are gone for good. They will be back and will bring others with them.

'My mother told me this and it is true. My daughter returned bringing a fiancé and my son returned with his two daughters.' – *Claire Vloedmans*

The best thing to give your child is your time.

'From my mum.' – *Ann Lusby*

To all first-time mothers, graciously accept all the advice you are given, then go away and do what *you* believe is best for your baby. Always remember that you know your baby better than anyone else does.

'I believe this came from my mother, when I was a young 18-year-old single mother. Everyone thought I needed their advice. When I became a grandmother, I told my daughters that I would give them unsolicited advice only once. But I would be available at all times if they wanted my help or advice.' – *Kerry Simmons*

Hug your children often. There is no such thing
as spoiling your babies with love and hugs.

'From my mum, when someone suggested that
picking up a crying baby was spoiling them.
Loving is not spoiling.' – *Judith Ferris*

If you don't want to get hurt, don't play with
your father.

'My dad was a prankster and lots of fun. He would
wrestle with us and chase us around the house and
was always scaring us.' – *Deslee Till*

Remember that your sons will someday be
husbands. Train them well.

'I was running around after my four- and six-year-
old sons, picking up toys, etc. Mum was visiting
and was just watching. When she told me this tip,
I stopped there and then. I was just doing what
was easier, I had never thought about my actions.
So by 10, they were stripping their beds for wash
day, remaking them, preparing veggies for dinner,
ironing their clothes, picking up after themselves.
About three times a year by age 13, they would look
for recipes and plan a week's worth of meals, then
check the cupboards for household needs within
a budget. We would shop together and I would
then cook the slow-cooker meats and freeze them.
They would defrost and make vegetables and salad
from their weekly planner. They happily stepped
in on occasion if I was late home from work and
they were hungry. My standards were higher than
my sons' so it wasn't easy – we had many tantrums,
tears, arguments and many times I wanted to just
do it myself, but Mum's words kept ringing in my
ears. Now as adults, they are very handy husband
material. Worth all the hassle and arguments.'
– *Nerilie Heikkinen*

A spoilt child is not a happy child.

'My mother gave me this piece of advice at some point when my two children were young. I can't remember the exact circumstances but would imagine it was some time when the kids were being particularly difficult and my mother obviously thought I was spoiling them. I found this advice invaluable as a parent.' – *Karen Rennick*

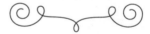

5 ways to boost confidence in shy grandkids

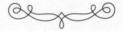

As grandparents, we all want to see our grandchildren happy and healthy. But if one of yours is suffering from severe shyness or a lack of confidence, how can you help bring them out of their shell?

The first step is to lead by example. So be warm to new people yourself, be polite to others and lend a helping hand when needed. Kids learn by watching the adults in their life, so model the ideal behaviour to them.

1. When meeting new people

Many kids clam up around new people, especially new adults. So take a moment to let them warm up before you introduce them. Get down on their level and let them know who the people are and how they fit in. It's also helpful if you give them a reason to believe this person can be trusted. For instance, 'This is Kate. Kate is my friend who lives next door. She has some chickens that we can go and visit sometime if you like?'

2. Visiting a shop or café

If your shy grandchild likes going out for a milkshake with you, encourage them to take charge of payment at the end. Have a practice at the table first so they know what to say. Then you can go to the counter and say, 'My grandson would like to pay the bill, please.' If it doesn't happen, it's not a big deal, but exposing them to these sorts of opportunities can be useful.

3. At an event
For children, a large gathering of people, such as a wedding, can be overwhelming. In the lead-up to it, advise what's going to happen and what's expected of them. For instance, 'At Joe's wedding, we'll sit down and have some lunch, and then you can go and play with your cousins in the garden.'

4. When dining out
Some shy children go beet-red when a waitress asks them what they'd like for dinner. While you don't want to force them to order if they don't want to, a great way to encourage them is to role-play at home beforehand. Play pretend restaurants and take their order on a notepad, letting them decide what they'll have from the menu. You could even have a look at the menu of the restaurant you're going to visit, so they can see what's on offer and what they might like to eat.

5. At a performance
If your grandchild is going to be in a school play or has to sing a song for Grandparents' Day, there's a good chance they'll be feeling nervous. Help them by reciting lines or practising the song together at home, where they feel most comfortable. You could let them know about a time when you felt shy or nervous but overcame it, and how wonderful it was to have been in the show with your friends.

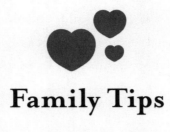

Family Tips

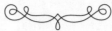

Always remember that your partner loves his/
her family as much as you love yours. So treat
them with as much respect and care as you would
your own.

'Advice given to me by my mother on my wedding
day.' – *Anita Kennedy*

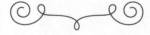

Don't ever expect your mother, lover, sister or another to make you happy. *You* are responsible for making you happy.

'My mother was responsible for my tip. It was part of her plan to raise her family to be resilient, to be thinkers, to be independent and self-sufficient if needed. It has stood me in good stead in many circumstances. I owe her a debt of gratitude.'
– *Del Dennis*

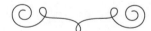

3 simple tips for a happier family

Nobody has the perfect family. We all have issues or difficult times that put the family dynamic under pressure. But there are things that you can do to try to improve the happiness levels in your family.

1. Talk about how you feel

Poor communication is often the tipping point for family breakdowns. Talking to each other lets your loved ones know how you're feeling. Feeling upset or angry with a family member isn't an excuse to shut off communication with them. In fact, you should now be sitting down to discuss how this makes you feel and find solutions. By ignoring the problem, it can fester into something bigger than it is. Don't forget to communicate about the positives, too – when someone has really helped you out or made you feel special. By letting them know that you notice and appreciate what they've done, you're encouraging more of the same behaviour down the track.

2. Listen to other people

Often we *think* that we're listening, but in fact we're just thinking about what we're going to say next, or wondering what's for dinner. To truly listen to someone, they need your full attention. You don't need to fix all their problems (if that's what they're talking about), just be attentive and empathetic. We all want to feel we're being heard. Listening without judgment shows respect to your family member.

3. Give and take

Remember that communicating with family is not about 'winning' an argument or always being right. Being able to compromise is important, as it shows there are ways to solve problems so that everyone wins.

Advice on dealing with tricky in-laws

There's nothing worse than heading to a family engagement when you have a son-in-law (or your daughter's parents-in-law) that you just don't get along with. From heated discussions to awkward family dinners, your relationship with your in-laws can have a big impact on family time. Here's how to navigate this sometimes-tricky dynamic, from those who have been there before.

1. Set boundaries

Do you know the old saying, 'good fences make good neighbours'? Think of your in-laws like your neighbours – you need to have really good 'fences' (boundaries) in place for the relationship to run smoothly. The best way to set boundaries is to ensure you don't make anyone feel you're shutting them out, but explain that you're focusing on yourself and things you have going on. Don't be afraid to talk to your family and in-laws about it; they're not as fragile as you think. But do choose your words carefully and keep the focus on you and what your needs are, rather than making judgments or comments about them or their behaviour.

2. Take a step back

The person you have the primary relationship with (i.e. your daughter, not your son-in-law) should be the one to step in and help fix a problem if it arises. You should never act as the messenger or go straight to an in-law. Gently raise the issue or concern with your immediate family member.

3. Limit contact

Decide what type of role you want your in-law/s to play in your life. If you don't get along and spending time with them just seems to cause issues, then you might want to limit catch-ups to birthdays and big events. This is okay. Just be gentle if pressed to explain. And keep your explanation brief and about you – something along the lines of, 'My schedule is quite busy at the moment,' or 'I don't feel up to going out much, but I am looking forward to the next family get-together.'

4. Keep the critical comments to yourself

Never criticise your family members for their relationship with their spouse or your in-laws. It's also important not to comment on your in-laws to your immediate family member. For example, don't criticise your son-in-law to your daughter/

his wife. This only leads to complications and awkwardness. And remember, you only know what your daughter tells you; if she comes to you whenever she's upset or angry with her partner or her partner's extended family, you're only hearing about problems when your daughter is frustrated and upset. You might not hear all the good things. Stay out of other people's arguments by reserving any judgment or comments.

5. Don't get involved

This is easier said than done. You have to trust you've brought your children up right and that they're responsible enough to navigate their own relationships, treat others respectfully and can stand up for themselves if need be. Their relationship issues, arguments and general day-to-day dealings are theirs, not yours. Stay on the peripheral, be there for some light guidance if need be but, ultimately, help them reach their own opinions, decisions and judgments on things rather than sharing yours with them.

6. Don't get sucked in

Don't get pulled into arguments by your child and in-laws.
Be supportive but let the couple handle their own problems.
Trust that you have raised an adult who has the vision and the
courage to resolve problems concerning their own family.
Couples need to set boundaries for their own relationships and
it can, as I'm sure you know, take time to find the right ones.

7. Think of yourself as a guest

When spending time in big family groups, and especially when
you're at someone else's home, it's best to think of yourself as
a guest and act accordingly. For example, you may not like
the way you son's wife is doing things in her home (child-
rearing, cooking, cleaning, etc.), but it's not really any of your
business. It's between your son and his wife. Ask yourself: Are
your expectations appropriate? If there are issues that you just
can't stand and can't let go, then you may need to consider not
visiting them.

A beginner's guide to starting a family tree

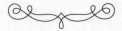

Keep the stories your grandparents told you alive by starting your own family tree. Along with birth dates and places, and the traditional elements of family trees, it's also a good place to document the tales your loved ones have passed down.

To research your family is to collect basic biographical details about the people in it. To do this, start with the events that are shared by everyone – birth and death. In many cases, marriage will also be on the list. After compiling these preliminary facts from legal or church records, you can then continue to build out other aspects of your family tree.

The Way Mum Does It

FIRST STEPS

Talk to family

When starting on your family tree, the first thing to do is talk to as many family members as possible, especially the older generations. This way, you can obtain the crucial first-hand accounts, memories and stories that will set you on your way. They can provide you with details of names, dates and key family events – although you should never take anything at face value, as it will be your job to investigate family myths. You may uncover skeletons in the cupboard as well – sometimes the most interesting part of your research.

Dig and delve

Now it's time to look through old family correspondence, photos, heirlooms and other material that can find its way into trunks, drawers, attics or cellars. You'll be amazed how much information you can extract from these objects to obtain vital clues as to who exactly your blood relations were, when they were born, who they married and who their children were. While doing this, be sure to note down any key figures in your family, as they will play an important role when you start looking further afield for relevant records.

GETTING STARTED

Visit a records office

You're now ready to pay a visit to an archive or records office – think state libraries or your local registry for births, deaths and marriages. Read the relevant leaflets and information available to you at the offices or on their websites. Start at the enquiries desk or the website's help/introduction section. Summarise who the person is and what information you want – be it a birth certificate, record of baptism or a will. This way, you should receive a much clearer answer than if you fall into the trap of recounting your entire family history. Just remember, there are usually fees involved for requesting information from such offices, as well as fees for document printouts.

Many records offices have compiled basic name indexes. Check these first, in case you uncover immediate references to an ancestor. Work backwards in time from known facts. Then use other catalogues and reference works to identify material that might contain information on relatives. Ask to see the original documents and work through them, hunting for information.

Seek out organisations and events

There are established professional organisations of genealogists with all levels of experience, or services such as Ancestry.com.au – a family history website that offers members access to 1 billion searchable Australian, New Zealand and United Kingdom family history records. Another resource is the Society of Australian Genealogists.

Family-history societies can also provide a ready-made support network of other genealogists working in your area. Most of these societies hold regular meetings and welcome new members. They hold activities and events, such as talks by members on their own research, visiting speakers and professional genealogists, and even excursions to record offices or other institutions.

Family-history fairs are another popular way of finding out more about genealogy. They are designed for researchers to meet representatives from major organisations. Many of the larger fairs are accompanied by lecture programs and are great fun for beginners looking for inspiration.

The best way to store family photos

Love the dog-eared, black-and-white photos of your grandparents and great grandparents? Ensure they're preserved for generations to come by adhering to best storing practices. Don't try to deny it. Somewhere in your home lies a box overflowing with weathered and faded family photographs, as well as scratched CDs holding hundreds of photos from recent years. Why let these treasured memories wither away or be corrupted? It only takes a few simple steps to save them from further deterioration and store them in a place for safekeeping, which won't take up precious space in your home.

Although photo restoration techniques have come a long way in recent years, don't be lulled into a false sense of security. It's far better to keep your valuable or treasured photos in prime condition from the start and to also house a digital backup. Digital storage solutions for photos are highly sophisticated, almost removing all need for physical storage at all. This means backing up your photos should become as natural as brushing your teeth. Remember, if you never off-load the images from your phone or camera, then your memories could be lost or damaged as easily as the device itself.

Even if you dutifully transfer your photos to a computer or website, you're not home free. Computers can crash or be destroyed in a disaster. Safeguard against the hazards of fate with two strategies: redundancy and geographic distribution. In other words, make multiple copies of photos and don't keep them all in the same place.

Store physical photos safely

Think of all those physical photos you don't have digital backups of. You should invest in a proper storage system. Your local craft store should have the basic supplies you'll need. Stock up on albums with archival sleeves and acid-free photo storage boxes.

Before filing and packing away old photos, remove and toss out paper clips, rubber bands, manila envelopes, staples and anything that has an odour. If your photos are stored in old albums you will want to remove them – especially the 'magnetic' or 'peel and stick' albums as the glue will damage photographs over time. If sorting large quantities of photos into boxes (choose 'acid free' cardboard or metal), pack each photo between acid-free paper. If storing individual photos in plastic sleeves, make sure they're 'PVC free'. Wear cotton gloves while handling old photographs to avoid long-term fingerprint damage.

Photos with historic significance should be treated extra carefully. In these cases, it's best to seek the help of a professionally trained conservator, who can clean, treat and prepare the photos for storage in the most effective manner possible.

For added safekeeping, consider scanning your print photo collection onto your computer.

Upload regularly

After an event or at a regular time each week, transfer photos from your camera or phone to your computer. It's a good idea to place photos in folders corresponding to the occasion or time frame (monthly, for instance), then keep those folders within a folder for that year. Copy the annual folder onto both an external hard drive and a cloud-storage service. That gives you two sets of backups for the photos on your computer.

Automate everything

Some photo-organising and image-editing software – Picasa, for example – will ask if it can scan your entire computer for photos. Once it's done, it displays all of the folders containing photos so you don't have to hunt for them. Alternatively, most external hard drives and online backup services include photo backup software. You can also use your operating system's backup utility. For Macs, it's called 'Time Machine'. For Windows, it's called the 'File History' feature in the Control Panel.

Cloud storage

Photos stored online are accessible no matter where you are. Cloud services usually offer limited space at no cost and charge for more. The options available include Dropbox, Microsoft OneDrive, Google Drive and Apple iCloud.

Tips for All Relationships

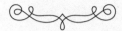

Be the best person you can be. Always be true to yourself, respect other people and their property, and always treat others as you would like to be treated yourself.

'Tips for life from my mum.' – *Patricia Margaret Longstaff*

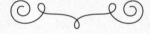

> Always listen to advice that's offered; try it and if it works, keep it, otherwise throw it out.

'My mum's advice came not long after I had my first child and I was drowning in the wisdom of all those well-meaning friends, parenting guides and the medical profession. I spent the first two weeks with Mum, learning how to survive having a newborn, and it was during that time she shared this piece of wisdom. I found it could be applied to all areas of life and have applied it successfully ever since. I have now passed it down to my daughter when she had her first-born child. My mum was my rock; she was always there, never interfering, just willing to listen and lend a hand. She passed away a few years ago but I still hear her wisdom coming through when I'm struggling with a problem or just enjoying the roses.'
– *Elizabeth Mace*

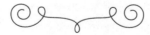

Mum always said to continue making friends throughout your life and make sure that some of them are much younger than you.

'She lived this advice her entire life – she died in 2016 at 91 – and she had friends in their twenties grieving her loss. It was a delight to see her energised and learning until the last week of her life, due to her contact with people of all ages and talents. She never stopped learning, smiling or making friends! I will follow her lead.' – *Dorothy Engelman*

If you can't say anything nice about someone, don't say anything at all.

'My mum gave me this advice when I was a teenager (I'm 67 now) and was gossiping about another teenager I heard about but didn't even know! It was a good lesson learnt, and I have passed it on to my children and grandchildren.' – *Lee Pattinson*

Love all. Trust a few. Always paddle your own canoe.

'My wise old mum wrote this in my autograph book in 1958 when I was just seven years old. At the time, I didn't really understand just what it meant, but as I grew and appreciated the wisdom of these words, I have tried to live my life like this. I have now passed it on to my four children and 13 grandchildren. I think this was her best life and parenting tip. Thank you, Mum.' – *Lynn McAuley*

Never put anything in writing that you wouldn't want someone else to read.

'I'm not sure where this came from. My mother gave me this advice when I was a teenager. I am now 64 years old and have followed this rule ever since.' – *Sue Harris*

How to disagree agreeably

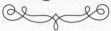

A disagreement doesn't have to devolve into an unsightly argument. Follow these six simple steps to disagree with respect.

1. Be calm

This is the most important thing you can do in this situation. A disagreement, even a simple one, can quickly cause emotions to become charged. That's when you'll start yelling, shouting insults and generally getting worked up. Take a deep breath, clear your mind and focus on what it is you want to say.

2. Stick to the facts

A respectful disagreement is one that focuses on logic, not emotion. Place your emphasis on reasoning and facts, rather than straying into subjective territory. You will also need to make sure your facts are correct, so be wary of taking someone to task on rumours or hearsay.

3. Be respectful

A disagreement is never one sided, so you'll need to listen to the other person's side of the story. If they feel that you are genuinely listening to them and hearing their opinion, they'll be more likely to think favourably of your side of the argument. And it goes without saying: yelling, making threats and using foul language are always off limits.

4. Use 'I' rather than 'you'

This simple language trick will prevent you from sounding too accusatory and confrontational. Try saying, 'I feel hurt when …' instead of saying, 'You hurt me when …' This should help to prevent the other person from getting on the defensive, while still allowing you to express how you feel.

5. Don't try to win

Your aim should be to reach a mutually agreeable resolution, not to score points. Try to focus on understanding what the other person has to say and on getting your own point across clearly. That way, you can clear the air and everyone can move forward feeling happy with the resolution.

6. Pick your battles

Disagreement is a part of life; don't feel the need to go into battle every time you have a difference of opinion. Take stock and decide if this issue is something you really care about, or if it would be easier for everyone if you just let it go. Sometimes silence is the best option for everyone.

Tips to get a relationship back on track

Sometimes a disagreement can spiral out of control. But an argument shouldn't spell the end of a relationship or friendship. Keep these tips in mind as you get things back on track:

- Give you and your partner time and space to process the argument. But at the same time, don't let things fester.

- Own your words by taking responsibility for what you said and did, even if you'd like to take it all back now.

- Don't keep bringing up what they said as the seed of future fights. And definitely don't share your argument on social media!

- Don't wait for your partner to say 'sorry' first, or be mean-spirited and not accept their apology straight away.

- Reaffirm your commitment to your friendship or relationship. But don't feel pressured into reconciling too soon if you're not ready.

'Resentment is like drinking a poison and then waiting for the other person to die.' – *Anonymous*

Never worry about what others may say about you, especially if it's nasty or mean. You know in your heart the kind and caring person you want to be; they still have to learn these life skills.

'This is what my mother told my daughter when she felt bullied at school.' – *Diane Thornton*

12 one-minute ways to boost relationships

It's the little things, not the big grand gestures, that keep a relationship ticking – and it doesn't take much to show your partner that you care and value them. These 12 tips each take less than a minute to do and, when you make a routine of these little ways to show love, they will instantly strengthen the bond in your relationship.

1. Surprise your spouse by doing an unpleasant or time-consuming task they normally do.

2. Plan to do something fun that you used to love doing together but stopped doing.

3. Thank your partner for something you usually take for granted.

4. Greet your partner with positivity and love first thing in the morning.

5. Compliment your partner. Let them know you love things about them they might not even like.

The Way Mum Does It

6. Bring up a fond memory of something you did together in the past.

7. Cuddle more.

8. Try a new way of expressing your love or bring back a nickname you've stopped using.

9. If you're apart for the day, send them a sweet text message or call to say you're thinking of them.

10. Ask them what's new and different in their lives (don't assume you already know everything there is to know!).

11. Do a project together.

12. Proclaim your love every day. It doesn't take much to tell your partner, 'I love you.'

4 steps to make friends anywhere

Making friends, like many social experiences, is a skill we learn. We learn how to form friendships as children, but may forget the skill as we grow older. We keep our friends as we move through our twenties and thirties and into middle age but, as we get into our more mature years, we may find friendships slipping away. This can lead to loneliness and isolation, without the connection and companionship we crave. Fortunately, making new friends isn't as intimidating as it sounds. Follow these four easy steps to make new friends, wherever you are.

1. Be alert and act interested.

When you're out and about, chat to the person making your coffee, or to the others waiting in line, especially if you think you might have something in common. Visit places where you might be able to meet like-minded people and take the first step. A smile and a simple question like, 'Do you come here often?' is a great start.

2. Listen to what they have to say.

If you're engaged in a conversation, pay attention! Enjoy chatting with your new friend and show interest in what they have to say.

3. Ask questions.

Don't be afraid to ask questions about your new friend. Nothing too intense: their favourite beverage (if you're at a café), where they like to eat in the area and similar questions help to build conversation and rapport.

4. Mention how much you've enjoyed chatting.

Leave the conversation at its natural conclusion. Then next time you see the person, chat to them again! You've started to build the foundations for a relationship and now you just need to be consistent.

5 tips for making social small talk

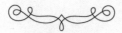

So often in life we find ourselves in a situation where we need to make some chit chat with a stranger or someone we don't know well. You might be at the bus stop, in the lunchroom at work, in a lift or at a small dinner party, and find yourself looking for something to say to break the silence. For some people this comes naturally, but for others it can be a stomach-churning experience that causes them to break out in a sweat. Here we have some easy-to-follow instructions for this type of situation, which will hopefully make small talk a little less awkward.

1. Remember your body language

Someone who is standing with good posture and a friendly face is always going to look more approachable than somebody with a slouch and a scowl.

2. Ask some open questions

The best way to get the conversation ball rolling is to ask open-ended questions – these are ones that can't be answered with a 'yes' or 'no'. For instance, you might say, 'I believe we're both friends with Kate. How do you two know each other?'

3. Add some humour

If the situation makes it appropriate, feel free to inject some humour into the conversation. But keep it light, and always beware that the decision to joke about someone else's poor taste in clothing or music could be met with 'That's my husband.'

4. Limit your life story

When you first meet someone, there's no need to start filling that person in on every unedited thought that goes through your head. Try to be interesting by focusing on topics such as a funny joke you heard, rather than telling them that you really need to remember to buy toilet paper on the way home.

5. Keep moving

If you try chatting to someone and it's not going anywhere, it's better to move on rather than battle on. Some people may also find small talk difficult, or maybe they're having a bad day and don't fancy striking up a conversation with you. You can say something like, 'Anyway, I'm off to the bathroom,' or 'I must just go and say hello to someone, would you excuse me?'

3 signs it's time to let go of a friendship

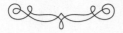

Friendships are one of life's most precious gifts. Your friends, some people say, are the family you choose for yourself. So it can be difficult to recognise when it's time to let some of those friendships go. Many people feel a sense of obligation to their friends – often labouring under the delusion that a friend is forever. The blunt truth of the matter: Not all friendships are built to last. A friendship might only have a shelf life of a year, a decade or even a single day. But it's important to remember never to assign blame when a friendship comes to a close.

Ending a friendship doesn't mean you wish this person ill, or never want to see them again, but it does mean that you want to take a step back and create some space in your life – either for yourself or for a new relationship. Let's look at some of the reasons you should be closing the chapter on a particular friendship.

1. Things have changed

Change is inevitable. Don't feel badly for admitting that something has changed – whether it's something in your life or theirs. Maybe you have changed, or perhaps your friend has. Maybe one of you has moved away, or started a new hobby, or begun a new job, or has entered a new relationship. Perhaps the thing you once had in common is gone. Whatever the change is, if it impacts the friendship, then you shouldn't feel guilty for recognising that shift and making the decision to move on from the friendship.

2. Too much work

A romantic relationship can be a lot of work – just about anyone will tell you this if you sit still long enough. But a friendship shouldn't be anywhere near as taxing on your energy – emotional or otherwise. If you feel you're pouring too much of your own energy into a friendship, then it might be time to pull back. This is especially true if you feel like your friend isn't contributing as much as you are. Again, it's important to remember that this is no one's fault.

3. Your needs aren't being met

Many of our friendships have specific purposes and functions – some of our friendships are built around the need to vent over coffee, or a shared passion for bargain hunting. Perhaps you are united by a love for romantic comedies, or of watching sports together. Whatever the commonality, if this is the strongest pillar upon which the friendship stands, then you can expect to feel a certain level of nourishment from that friendship. If, however, circumstances change and you're no longer having those specific needs met, it might be time to call it quits.

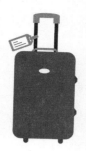

Travel

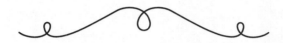

'Be sure to travel. Work, including housework, will always be there, but the chance to see the world might not. My mum had always dreamed of travelling through Britain and we did that as a family when I was eight years old. A couple of years later we lost everything, and then a few years after that my father passed away. Mum never got the chance to return and explore all those country lanes she'd wanted to see again. Her motto, therefore, has always been to "seize the day."'

— *Sheriden Rhodes, travel writer and photographer*

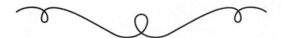

Planning Tips

Peak travel times are guaranteed to cost more, wherever you're going. If you can be flexible, avoid peak summer, school holidays or holiday seasons like Christmas. Airlines and hotels charge top dollar when demand is high. Shoulder season – just before the start of, or just after the end of, peak season – is a better option. You'll get many of the benefits of peak season but at a much lower cost.

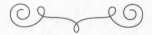

When planning for a holiday, the first thing to do is make a list. A big one. On it, you should include everything that needs to be done before your holiday, from booking the tickets and buying travel insurance to asking a loved one or friend to check on your home periodically while you're away. Keep this as an ongoing task list for a few weeks before you travel and, every time you think of something else, add it to the list. This will help to ensure you remember everything important that needs to be done and will ease the anxiety of feeling like you've missed something. And one last tip with planning: send a copy of all of your travel documents to someone at home, just in case of an emergency.

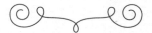

Plan ahead! Organise the outfits you pack so you maximise the number of wears possible from each item. Think staples like jeans, trousers, wear-anywhere blouses that double for day and night outings, and a smart blazer. You'll also want to pack clothing in solid or neutral colours that mix and match well. Scarves/shawls/sarongs make versatile accessories. If you can only wear something once and it doesn't go with two or three other items, leave it behind.

There are lots of things to check off before you travel – some pretty standard, some particular to your circumstances. Obviously having people back home looking after your house, contents and car is a big bonus but, if you'll be away for six months, there are additional concerns, such as deflating your car tyres and rotating the wheels, organising someone to mow the lawn or rake up autumn leaves, or cleaning out and unplugging the fridge.

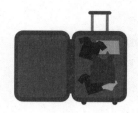

Packing Tips

Before packing, make a list of your essentials for the trip. Then cross them out as you pack. Keep the list for future trips and add or delete items over time. You'll have a peaceful night's sleep before you go – as you won't be thinking about what you've forgotten.

'This came from regularly lying down to go to sleep and getting up every 10 minutes when something else came to mind. Now all I have to do is cut back on the superfluous things that aren't used each time.'
– *Leonard Byrne*

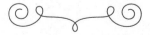

If travelling with a companion, put half of your clothes in their bag and vice versa. That way, if one of your bags get lost you'll still have some clothes until you can buy more.

A neat way to carry around travel documents is money belts, as they're generally pretty discreet. Strapped around your stomach, they let you keep your important travel documents on your person without running the risk of them being nabbed by pickpockets. That said, money belts are only so big; they might not be suitable for all of your travel documents.

With your planning organised and perfected and well-thought-out outfits packed, it's time to throw caution to the wind. It's a holiday, after all. While it's natural to be a tad nervous about having new experiences and exploring new places, you've done the hard yards to get away; leave room for the unexpected. Part of the joy of being so organised is being able to take time out when you're there. From cruising down the Thames on a boat to getting lost in a bustling marketplace, whatever opportunity comes your way, try and experience as much as you can while you're on holiday. And don't forget to take pictures!

5 clever ways to organise cables while travelling

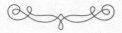

It's quite alarming to think about all the minutes (or even hours) of our lives we've wasted untangling cables attached to our earphones, electronics and charging devices. When you're living out of suitcases and on the move, those cords seem to get in even more of a tangle. The good news is, with a bit of prep, you can keep cables organised without having to invest in expensive travel gear. Here are five of our top tips.

1. Old glasses case
Perfect if you want to protect your cable from the elements, an old, unused glasses case provides durable, waterproof protection. Your cable will remain in place, protected from damage and any unnecessary tangling.

2. Bendable twist ties
If you're confident your cable won't be damaged, a bendable twist tie is a great option. At a pinch, you could even use one from a loaf of bread (although it won't be as sturdy as purpose-bought ties).

3. Sandwich bags

If you're after waterproof protection for your cables, a small zip-lock sandwich bag is a decent solution. These are easily opened and sealed, ensuring your cable will remain undamaged by elemental forces, untangled and ready to use.

4. Used toilet-paper rolls

The practicalities of used toilet-paper rolls have no bounds. Cut a notch at each end of the tube's rim and wrap your cable around inside, securing the plug ends in the new grooves. You'll wonder how you ever travelled without them!

5. Bulldog clips

They might seem out of place outside an office, but bulldog clips are ideal to keep cords untangled and organised. Clip them inside your bag (or even to your shirt) and you can be sure that your cords will remain in order and in place.

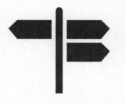

On the Road Tips

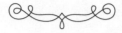

Always be careful when drinking and never leave drinks unattended or in the care of a stranger or new friend.

Use only officially licensed and reputable taxis to get around. Beware of people posing at taxi drivers – they usually try to accost you at tourist hotspots.

When on the road travelling, place your dirty laundry in a large bucket (which has a tight-fitting lid) with water and washing powder. Place it on the floor of your caravan, trailer or car boot, make sure the lid is firmly closed, and the vibrations from the road as you're driving will wash your clothes cleaner than a machine. When you get to your destination, rinse in clean water and hang out to dry. Saves time in a Laundromat, is much cheaper and requires less work than hand-washing. Big plastic rubbish bins with clip-on lids are great for sheets and towels, and can be re-used for storage when they're not being used as mini washing machines.

'I learned this tip from a fellow traveller who'd been "on the road" for 18 months. She even re-used the soapy water to wash down the car and caravan.'
– *Greta Dabrowski*

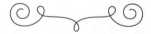

How to be water-wise overseas

Part of the reason so many people have fallen sick after drinking water overseas is the fact that they were blissfully unaware of the risks that were posed. Make sure you research your destination and figure out if water quality is going to be a problem on your trip.

Along with always having bottled water for drinking:

- Use bottled water for cleaning teeth.
- Avoid ice cubes in your drink as they could be made with local water.
- Steer clear of salad as the leaves were probably washed in local water.
- And don't forget to keep your mouth closed in the shower!

6 essential tips for travelling with kids

Spending time with kids can be both a rewarding and frustrating experience. While they can be an infinite source of cuddles and homemade artwork, little ones can also bring out the worst in us, leading to family arguments and the testing of even the strongest relationships. So if you are planning a trip with little ones, here's how to make the most of the opportunity for a family holiday.

1. Get their input

Rather than just planning everything out for them, ask their help to decide on the itinerary. By being involved in the decision-making process, they'll feel more of an equal player on the trip. They are also less likely to make a fuss when you let them know it's time to go to the museum now, even when they're having fun in the pool.

2. Lay out the ground rules

Let the little ones know what's going to happen in terms of who pays for what. This could be theme park entries, souvenir purchases, or meals and snacks. This should eliminate issues down the track.

3. Decide on 'fair use' for electronic devices

While you may not be obsessed with your smartphone, tablet,
gaming console or laptop – your children or grandchildren
might be. Allow them to use their devices for at least a short
time each day on your trip, but for grandchildren, first check
with their parents on the family rules. Feel free to put your own
rules in place, too, such as no devices during meal times.

4. Allow for changes of plan

Don't be too rigid with your schedule as kids can, of course,
be unpredictable with their moods. If you notice the kids are
getting tired or emotional, it might be a good idea to skip a
planned activity in favour of more down time or some time
apart. Older children might want to make an unscheduled
stop, based on a recommendation from someone they meet on
the trip. Always take their ideas on board rather than outright
dismissing them, and opt for a group consensus if it will
affect everyone.

5. Plan for relaxation time

Allow for down time each day, as being on the go can be exhausting for kids, parents and grandparents alike. Build this into your schedule, whether that means naps for little ones, watching movies or just relaxing by the pool.

6. Make your own memories

When things go wrong or the weather is bad, consider it an opportunity rather than a disaster. Use these times to talk to the kids about times when your travel plans have gone awry and led to a fun or interesting outcome. Purposely take part in activities that you know they'll remember as they grow older – it could be trying a fun new food together, sleeping under the stars, trekking up a mountain to watch the sunset, or getting up early to go fishing on the beach together.

6 ways to keep your data safe while travelling

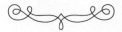

Data thieves are the modern-day pickpockets. Here's how to keep your data safe while you're on holiday.

1. Be wary of public Wi-Fi

A free, open Wi-Fi network can seem like a great find – here's your chance to get online for nothing! But make sure it's a reputable source, such as from a hotel, city council or restaurant. Unscrupulous types can easily set up these networks and, once you've logged on, quickly swipe your data. If you don't recognise the name, it's best to stay away.

2. Think before you type

If you're not sure about the security of a Wi-Fi network, don't put in any of your sensitive information. That means banking details, credit card numbers or even passwords. Save these for when you know you can trust your connection.

3. Protect your privacy

Most smartphones and tablets have location settings built into their apps. This means that every time you update your status, log in or take a picture, your precise location is recorded and (sometimes) published. This kind of info can be useful to cyber criminals, so the safest thing to do is switch them off. Go into your settings and look under 'Privacy'.

4. Stay alert

Sadly, most people aren't scammed through some high-tech trickery – they hand over their own information. Suspicious emails, pop ups, phishing scams and more will appear in your inbox or on your screen and ask for your details. Usually, they will claim you've won a prize or can access some special content, but be wary. If things sound too good to be true, they generally are. Unless you are 100 per cent sure, don't enter any information.

5. Stay up to date

Before you travel, make sure all operating systems and anti-virus software are up to date on your smartphone, tablet or computer. These programs are your first line of defence against hackers, so if you're behind the times you've left yourself vulnerable. You should also employ the best security options available, such as fingerprint recognition or passcodes.

6. Back up regularly

If the worst does happen and someone manages to hack your data, you don't want to lose everything. It makes sense to regularly back up your photos and significant data on an external hard drive. That way, you have a second copy that will stay safe and out of reach of anyone who shouldn't be looking.

The 5 best ways to save photos while travelling

Gone are the days when you'd take roll after roll of film on holiday then wait in excitement at the photo developer's for your prints to come out. And the choices: Do you get a white border? 3 x 5 inch or 4 x 6 inch prints?

These days you can curate your holiday snaps as you go. Just remember not to spend your whole holiday behind the lens – some of your best experiences will be when you put your camera or phone away. You'll never lose a moment again with these handy tips for saving or sharing your digital photos while you're on the road.

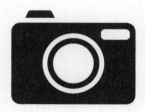

1. Email

This is the simplest, easiest way to save a copy of your pictures online. Email them to yourself or to a friend, then download them when you're ready. It's also an easy way to keep your contacts up to date with your travels. However, you'll need to think about the size of the files you're sending. Some digital cameras will give you an option to create smaller files suitable for emailing, or you can downsize them yourself on a computer.

2. Cloud

Store all your images safely online in a remote database or 'the cloud'. There are a number of free and paid services available that allow for the quick and easy upload of large numbers of files at once, provided you have a good internet connection. These include Dropbox, Google Drive, Apple iCloud or Amazon Cloud Drive.

3. Sharing service

These sites will let you both store and share your photos in one easy move. Flickr is the most popular and allows you to create a free page for yourself, where you can upload multiple images divided into galleries. You can then send the link to your friends and family so they can see your holiday snaps. Even your own Facebook page is a good spot to keep images; you can control the privacy settings to restrict who has access.

4. Personal website

It's easy to create your own personal website. Use it as a place to store your images, share them with friends and post blog updates about your travels. Simple blogging sites, such as WordPress, are free and can be customised to suit your needs. Create a record of your travels in an easy-to-use format that preserves your photos safely online.

5. Hardware

If you'd prefer to have a physical backup of your photos, then look into additional memory cards or a portable hard drive to take with you. You can download a huge number of photos onto a relatively small drive, then transfer them to your computer when you get home. The one thing to be careful of is losing the device itself – because the photos exist only on the physical drive, there is no online backup.

10 ways to enjoy food on holidays without putting on weight

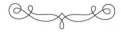

One of the best (or at least tastiest) parts of an overseas holiday is all the incredible food you get to try. But, if you're not careful, you might be coming home with some excess baggage (in more ways than one). Here are 10 tips for enjoying food while you're on holidays, so you can experience incredible international cuisines without putting on weight.

1. Pack your own food when in transit

Whether you're travelling by plane, ferry, bus or car, packing your own food will help you resist the temptation to buy high-fat fast food. You'll also save a small fortune.

2. Once you arrive, stock up on healthy snacks

As soon as you get to your destination, head to the local supermarket and pick up a few healthy snacks that you can enjoy between meals or while exploring.

3. Plan your days to avoid overeating

Planning a long leisurely lunch? Try to have a smaller dinner. Heading to a buffet in the evening? Choose a light lunch. Plan ahead, and make sure you don't skip meals.

4. Be strategic with your breakfast

Breakfast can really set your metabolism up for the day, so be strategic when partaking in the most important meal of the day. Opt for something that will keep you full.

5. Try (if possible) to avoid carbs after 6 p.m.

Eating at later times is often common on holidays, but this can be bad for your metabolism. Stick to those pasta and rice dishes for lunch if dinner will be a late one.

6. Don't overdo it on the rich dishes

Anything fried, sautéed, flambéed or roasted is bound to taste good, but is also likely to have been cooked with oil. Try not to overdo it with the rich dishes.

7. Do your sightseeing on foot

Instead of opting for a car or bus tour, do your sightseeing on foot. Not only will this burn kilojoules, you'll also get a much better look at the attraction.

8. Go easy on the booze

Sure, we all like to partake in a drink (or three) while on holidays, but excessive alcohol can lead to us snacking later. So try to go easy on the booze on your trip.

9. Take an evening stroll

You're on holidays so there's no reason to get up early in the morning! An evening stroll is the perfect way to enjoy a beach or explore the nearest town.

10. Don't completely deprive yourself

At the end of the day, however, you have to remember that you're on holidays. Don't be afraid to enjoy your food and drink, as long as you're enjoying everything in moderation.

How to avoid deep vein thrombosis while travelling

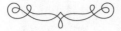

Generally occurring in your leg, deep vein thrombosis (DVT) is a serious condition where a blood clot forms in one of your deeper veins. In minor cases, DVT causes pain and uncomfortable swelling, and can even lead to serious health complications. Any form of travel that has you seated in the one position for an extended period increases your risk of DVT, whether you're travelling by car, bus, train or air. Here are some simple measures you can take when travelling to avoid DVT and make sure you remember your holiday for the right reasons.

Stand up and move around

Sitting in a position where your leg is bent for an extended period of time significantly reduces blood flow and increases your risk of a clot. Something as simple as standing every now and then to walk up and down the aisle of the bus, train or plane can really help your circulation. And if you're driving, stop every couple of hours for a quick stroll.

Compression socks

If you have a history of DVT, it might be an idea to invest in some fitted compression socks. These useful leggings help to improve the blood flow in your lower legs. Compressions socks

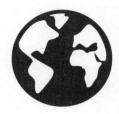

are available in a variety of different sizes so you can choose the best one to suit your circumstances, depending on where you suffered blood clots in the past.

Blood-thinning medication

This is for more serious cases, of course, but if you're highly concerned about the occurrence of DVT on your next trip, consider asking your doctor for blood-thinning medication prior. This medication will generally reduce your blood's ability to clot while travelling, while at the same time preventing existing clots from becoming bigger.

Stay hydrated

Dehydration can significantly increase your risk of coming down with DVT. This causes your blood volume to decrease and 'thicken', significantly increasing the likelihood of a clot occurring. Make sure you drink plenty of water while you're on your trip and be mindful about the alcohol you're consuming, as that can lead to dehydration.

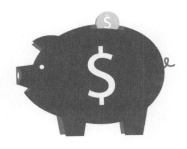

Finances

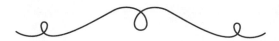

'My father always said, "If you divided up all the money in the world and gave each person an equal share, it would be back in the same hands within a week." He also said, "If you do one good turn, you get two good turns back." And my grandfather said, "I don't smoke – I couldn't bear the thought of watching my money going up in smoke."'

— Noel Whittaker, AM, financial expert and author

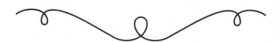

These tips are for general advice only and should not be relied on as financial advice. You should consider seeking formal advice about your specific circumstances.

My mum always told me to look after the cents and the dollars would look after themselves.

'Growing up, I wanted a bike and that is what she told me to do. I got my bike.' – *Kay Rose*

If you have limited space for a filing cabinet, a good system is a hard A4 folder to file bills and documents. Go through them once a year for a clear out.

Budget to cover expected bills by saving something each week.

'During my childhood in the 1950s, my mother used to have a row of Vegemite jars (the ones that could be used as a glass, or container, if the lid was kept). Every payday, when my father came home with his envelope of cash, she'd put some coins into each jar so that when the gas or electricity bill (or any other expected bill) came in, the money would be available to pay the account. As I watched, I learnt how to budget. To this day, I've never had a problem with overdue accounts because my mother taught me how to save regularly for the expected, with a spare jar for the unexpected.' – *Shirley McDermott*

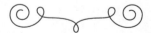

5 things money-wise people never do

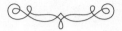

Your mother or grandmother probably warned you how easy it is to fall prey to hidden service fees, slick marketing hype and sneaky sales pitches. Here are a few tips to steer clear of some typical financial pitfalls, stamped with Mother's approval.

1. Don't get lured by the clearance sale signs

For those with a head for money, getting a bargain is thrill. But, just because something is cheap doesn't make it a bargain if you don't need it and won't use it. Think carefully about what you'll do with that heavily discounted item before you make the purchase.

2. Steer clear of full-price household items

Waiting until end-of-season sales ensures you can stock up on wardrobe essentials, without breaking the bank. There's nothing more annoying after buying a suit than seeing it half price a week later! You can purchase furniture and white goods from factory outlets or auction websites, or ask sales assistants about floor stock that may be slightly marked but heavily discounted. Also, don't be afraid to ask (especially when making a big purchase) whether the advertised price is the best they can do, and to request a discount for multiple purchases. You may be surprised how far they're willing to go for your business.

3. Do your research before buying big-ticket items

Many large stores price match (even if they don't advertise it) because they want to keep your business. Before you make a big purchase, ensure you research the product. In the old days, word-of-mouth ruled, but today there are plentiful reviews on product comparison sites.

4. Pay that interest on your credit card

Money-smart people don't have credit card debt that can't be paid off each month. Minimise the number of credit cards you have (one is usually enough to do things like internet purchases) and make sure you get one that works for you. Perhaps pick one with an interest-free period, or one that allows you to earn points and pay off the balance in full each month. Or, better yet, if you know you might struggle to pay it off, ditch the credit card altogether and use a debit card instead.

5. Resist buying that brand-new car

There's a saying that you lose money on a new car even as you drive it out of the yard, because cars depreciate in value very quickly. Buying a near-new second-hand car or a demonstration vehicle means you get a lot more bang for your buck. You'll pay less buying through a private seller than a dealer, but make sure you enquire about the reasons for selling and check that the car doesn't have finance owing, and that it hasn't been in any accidents, before you commit to buying.

20 small ways to reduce your monthly spend

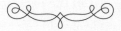

During wartime, our mothers and grandmothers practically perfected ways to live on less. Even though you might try your best to budget, sometimes it can seem as though the exact same amount of money is going out as what's coming back in. The good news is that saving needn't necessarily be so hard. We've outlined 20 small but effective ways to reduce your average monthly spend. Follow these expert tips and we're sure you'll notice plenty of extra spare change in your wallet when it gets to the end of the month.

1. Install energy-efficient LED light bulbs

LEDs use even less power than CFLs (compact fluorescent lights), and are a fraction of the wattage of old-fashioned incandescent bulbs. Electricity rates certainly aren't getting any cheaper, and it really pays to try and save wherever you can.

2. Unplug unused electrical devices

When some electrical devices are plugged in, they continue to drain power so, when you're not using your devices, pull the plug out and save.

3. Opt for inexpensive entertainment

If you're spending a king's ransom keeping yourself entertained, consider cheaper options, such as visiting your local library.

4. Cancel unused subscriptions

You may love the thud of a newspaper on your front step in the morning, but if you're not actually reading it, it's an unnecessary expense.

5. Cook more meals at home

There's nothing wrong with eating out occasionally but when this becomes a major habit, it can have a big impact on your back pocket.

6. Start a vegetable garden

Don't leave yourself at the mercy of supermarkets and green grocers. Starting a vegetable garden is a great hobby and an even better way to get fresh produce.

7. Buy generic items

We've all got our favourite brands, but that label does come with a premium. And in many cases, the generic option is really just as good.

8. Shop around for cheaper phone plans

So many people are paying more than they have to because they're getting overcharged or just haven't looked around.

9. Go easy on the booze

Everybody likes a drink every now and then, but this can be an expensive habit. Going dry a couple of days a week will make your wallet (and liver) thank you.

10. Buy non-perishables in bulk

Often you can secure pretty reasonable prices for non-perishable items when buying in bulk. Simply freeze and eat when you're ready.

11. Shop around insurance policies

It might be time to consider your level of coverage. Talk to your provider and others to see if you're currently over-insured. Insurance companies may be hitting you with a 'lazy tax' – by offering special deals and incentives to win over new customers but not extending these to existing customers, your loyalty may be costing you – so annually, it's a good idea to shop around to see if another provider offers you an incentive to switch.

12. Make your own gifts

At the end of the day, it's the thought that counts. So if you've got a loved one with a special occasion coming up, consider making your own gift.

13. Never shop on an empty stomach

Research has shown that showing up to a supermarket hungry makes shoppers more likely to make impulse buys.

14. Consider second-hand clothes

Buying new outfits all the time can add up, so if you need a woolly sweater try going to an op-shop. You may pick up a barely worn designer purchase for a fraction of the retail price!

15. Wait 30 days before making a major purchase

You might feel as though you want to buy something, but wait 30 days to see if that urge is still there.

16. Entertain guests at home instead of going out

Going out all the time can be quite expensive; inviting your friends over to your place ends up much cheaper.

17. Refillable water bottles

Bottled water is one expense that is never really justified, especially when you consider how much cheaper it is to buy a refillable bottle.

18. Stop smoking

Cutting out smoking is probably the single best way to make you healthier and save some money.

19. Turn off lights when you're not in the room

So often we leave the lights on in the house out of habit but, if no one's in the room, you're just wasting money.

20. Skip the café coffee

Buying coffee can be expensive if you do it every day. If you skip it for homemade options, you can save hundreds each year.

Top tips for avoiding money scams

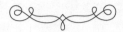

Financial scammers have been trying to cheat hardworking parents and grandparents since before Charles Ponzi and his infamous pyramid scheme. With technology evolving and more people going online to pay bills, communicate with friends and family, and even find love, some unwitting and unlucky people have sent money overseas or elsewhere never to see it again. Falling victim to a clever scam artist is something we all fear! With these top tips, we show you how to avoid getting ripped off.

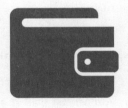

What to look out for

Financial fraud can come in any form. It can be an email from a stranger asking for a donation to a charitable cause, or a phone call promising a once-in-a-lifetime investment opportunity. However, as the saying goes, if it sounds too good to be true, it's because it probably is.

According to the Australian Competition and Consumer Commission's (ACCC) SCAMwatch site – a one-stop information shop on how to recognise, avoid and report scams – almost everyone will be approached by a scammer at some stage in their life. That's a scary pronouncement, but one that's very much evident in the growing number of stories of people who have fallen victim to a scam.

While some scams are easy to spot, others appear to be genuine offers or bargains. There are a number of different types of scams, too, from investment and superannuation scams to those involving your bank or credit card. It can even look as innocent as a supermarket customer satisfaction survey.

Warning signs

Scams can target people of all backgrounds, ages and income
levels. The reason many people fall victim to a scam is because
they look like the real thing. It could look like a legitimate
business email or letter, with logos, contact details and genuine
information that could be targeting a specific need or desire.
It's not until you dig a little deeper that you find something
isn't right.

Scammers can also manipulate you by 'pushing your buttons',
according to the ACCC, to get an automatic response. This is
not based on you personally but on how society works as a whole.
It's not until after you've acted in the way they want that you find
something is wrong.

The best way to spot a scam is to be vigilant and cautious,
especially when it comes to giving out personal details over
the internet or the phone. Most scams will need you to do
something before they can work. They may ask for your bank
or credit card details, or for you to send them money based on
the promise of a significant financial reward that turns out to
be false. Some scams also rely on you to agree to deals without
getting advice first, or to buy a product without properly looking
into it.

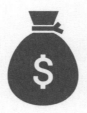

Don't be a victim

The first step in protecting yourself against scams and other forms of financial fraud is to be aware that it *can* happen. Some people hold certain perceptions that make them more susceptible to being scammed, such as the belief that all companies or organisations are legitimate or that all internet sites are legitimate. Both are myths.

Consumer protection agencies try to weed out dodgy operators before they have an impact, but sometimes one can slip through the net. Most of these fake sites will be taken down after a few days, but that is still long enough for someone to buy into a dodgy deal or provide their bank details to a scammer.

The second step is to be cautious and protective of your personal details. This includes your contact details and bank or credit card details. Always seek independent advice before agreeing to any sort of money commitment and remember, there are no get-rich-quick schemes. Check your bank statements regularly and if you see a transaction that you're not sure about or cannot explain, contact your bank or credit union. Also, keep your bankcards and personal identity number (PIN) safe and secure.

Be cautious and question everything. It's the best approach to make sure you don't become a scam victim.

How to save for a rainy day

Just like many grandparents and parents have advised, it's important to be prepared for life's unexpected moments. You may have to make an interstate trip on short notice, or your employer has gone kaput and let go its workers. Having spare money on hand to dip into for emergencies can take the stress out of these unexpected times.

The trick to setting up a 'rainy day' fund is to put small amounts of money away on a regular basis (and not taking a sneaky dip into it now and then!) Over time, this will add up and your future self will thank you for the effort.

Where to start?

When it comes to how much you stash away in your emergency fund, this will all depend on your weekly budget. A small amount of $10 per week could be a good start. Over 12 months, this will amount to more than $500. You can always put away more as you review your budget; see what works for you.

The other way to come up with a monetary goal for your emergency fund is to estimate the costs of expenses, such as medical bills or a short-notice flight to where your family live.

Add these together and whatever dollar figure you get, aim to save up to that amount. From here, take a look at your weekly budget and see how you can regularly top up your emergency fund to meet this monetary goal.

Where should I put it?

If you plan on putting money into your emergency fund on a regular basis, consider opening a high-interest savings bank account. This way you can earn interest on the cash you put in there and help it grow quicker. Some of the best rates are available only on high-interest online savings accounts, so you'll need to apply and manage the money entirely online.

If you're not comfortable with online banking, go into your local bank branch and ask them about their interest rates for a savings account. Ask about the account's fees and other conditions as well, since you don't want all of your money eaten up by bank charges.

And if you have a healthy distrust of banks, you could always go with the trusty piggy bank or money jar kept hidden in a safe place.

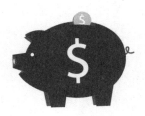

Help with budgeting

There are a number of apps available for smartphones and tablets, which can help you to manage your expenses to save. Apps such as Pocketbook help you to coordinate all of your bank accounts into the one area so you can track your spending. If you're someone who makes a lot of transactions during the week, it can be handy having an app to help you record where your money is going. Budgeting apps have become really popular because they can save you a lot of money, just by letting you know where your money is going. When it comes to saving for an emergency fund, a budgeting app may be able to help you cut back on spending in one area, like takeaway coffee, and to put that money into your emergency fund.

Many people think there's no money in their budget to fork out regular payments, no matter how small. But you'd be surprised. Take a glance at your expenses in one week and have a think about where you can redirect some cash you won't miss too much into an emergency fund. Start small and see where you progress; you may be pleasantly surprised.

Here are four other tips for getting your rainy-day fund in tip-top shape right now:

1. Save your small change

Pay for groceries and expenses with notes (if you have them handy) and set aside all of your coins. At the end of each month, divide them into different coin bags and deposit them at the coin counters of your local bank branch.

2. Get smart with your leftovers

After withdrawing a certain amount each week from the ATM, place whatever you don't use at the end of the week into a jar. We all love a bit of healthy competition, so see how much you can cut into your weekly expenses to make your rainy-day jar just that little bit heavier each week.

3. Out of sight, out of mind

On payday, set up an automatic bank transfer of $20 to $50 (whatever you think you can spare on a regular basis) from your everyday account to a high-interest savings account. By doing this automatically, you'll never see what money you have to spend each week or month. After three to six months, review your budget to see if you can possibly get away with adding more to your automatic transfers.

4. Keep cash hidden from yourself

When there is a $20 or $50 note sitting in your wallet, chances are it's going to be spent (unless you're really self-disciplined). If you're going shopping and don't trust yourself not to spend it, hide the extra note or two in a side pocket of your wallet. If you can't 'see' it, you can't spend it! At the end of the month, see how much is stashed away in your little side pocket and pop it in your rainy-day fund. Instant windfall!

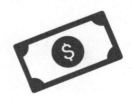

5 simple tricks to reduce your energy bill in winter

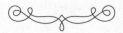

Winter is a time when we love to hibernate at home and stay toasty warm, but the impact on the electricity bill can be enormous. From rugging up with the blanket your grandma knitted to checking the seals around your home, here are five smart ways to stay warm and reduce the chill on your hip pocket.

1. Rug up

An easy way to save electricity and stay warm in winter is to put on suitable clothing. A big woolly jumper, warm pants and indoor slippers are not only comfortable for relaxing around the home, they'll also keep you toasty warm. While you don't have to resort to wearing a big overcoat or winter jacket inside your home, it's a good idea to put on an extra couple of layers and save having to switch on the heater. However, don't endure being cold for the sake of not putting on your heater. Find what works for you, as long you're comfortable and warm.

2. Seal your home

Chilly draughts from poorly sealed windows and doors are a nuisance and can also account for a big percentage of the heat loss from naturally insulated rooms or the heater. Keep the heat inside by sealing any gaps and cracks in external walls, floors and the ceiling. Seal external doors with draught stoppers or those classic door snakes at the bottom of doors, and install weather stripping around the frames.

3. Load up on blankets

Who needs an electric blanket when you can add any number of layers to your bed? Call them duvets, doonas, quilts or comforters, just keep layering until your bed is a warm haven. For the same instant warmness as an electric blanket, heat a hot water bottle and pop it between the sheets just before you go to bed. While it won't heat the entire bed evenly, it makes the bed feel warmer while your body adjusts to the enclosed space.

4. Let the sun in

Winter can sometimes offer up a surprise in the form of a clear blue sky and some warming sunlight. When it does, open up the windows and doors (if there's no cool breeze) and allow the sun's rays to heat your home naturally. Just remember to close everything up as soon as the warmth begins to go.

5. Shop around for energy providers

This is the best way to make sure you're getting a good deal on your energy usage. Depending on what state you live in, you should be able to find a range of energy retailers offering competitive prices for their services.

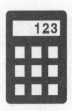

Money and Finance Tips

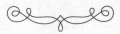

You don't have to look far to find someone who is worse off than yourself.

'My mother was a practical person. She taught my sisters and me to make the best of what we had, so if we wanted something that was unattainable, we would not be disappointed.' – *Val Power*

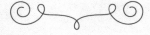

Check your credit card interest rate and charges – you may be paying way more than you should. Shop around, then try calling your credit card company to negotiate a better rate.

Got a gym membership you rarely use? Cancel it and save! Hunt around for second-hand gym equipment (Gumtree and eBay are two useful websites), find workout videos online, or use household items like full cans and drink bottles as free weights.

5 super-simple ways to save money for retirement

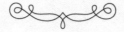

During the lead-in to retirement, money management becomes more important than ever. And while we often get lost pondering over the major financial decisions, getting the minor financial decisions right can be just as important.

We're going to run through five simple ways any soon-to-be-retiree can save cash for their golden years. Sometimes the smallest changes make the biggest difference.

1. Set targets

Saving can be difficult if you don't know where the goalposts are placed. But how much do you really need to retire? The Association of Superannuation Funds of Australia says that a couple needs approximately $640,000 in retirement savings for a comfortable lifestyle. A single person needs around $545,000. Setting minor saving targets, even if it's just a little bit of money here and there every week, can get the ball rolling.

2. Shop smarter

While you don't want to be living like a miser, smarter shopping choices can add up. Keep your ear to the ground for discounts, take advantage of specials and avoid unnecessary purchases to help keep you in the black and start putting yourself in a position to prop up your nest egg.

3. Clear any outstanding debt

Debt can be an inconvenient drain on your income in the lead-in to retirement. If you're set to take the plunge and find yourself in a mire of debt, it's important to take necessary steps as soon as possible. Consider talking to a financial planner about how best to clear your debts.

4. Change spending habits

Ultimately, if you're looking to save some extra cash for retirement, you're going to have to change your spending habits. Little things like drinking coffee at home, or staying in for lunch and dinner, can make a big difference in the long run.

5. Explore your options

Taking the measures listed above is a good start, but you're only scratching the surface of what you can do to prop up your retirement income. Qualified financial planners can give you advice and guidance on things you can do in your day-to-day life that will ensure you're in a better financial position when you've reached retirement.

Make do and mend — go back to basics to save money

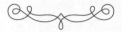

When the story of the current zeitgeist comes to be written, it might well be captured in a four-word slogan that defined the spirit of wartime Britain. Part admonition, part joyful declaration of intent, 'Make Do and Mend' became the catch-cry of a generation that kept calm and carried on through the darkest days of World War II.

The British Ministry of Information adopted this campaign slogan as it recommended everything from how to grow vegetables, reuse leftovers and make new clothes from old. Nimble fingers unpicked and reknitted woolen jumpers, upcycled government-issue blankets into skirts and jackets, and raised cabbages and carrots in municipal flowerbeds.

Today, as the world confronts fresh environmental and economic hardships, it's time to heed the lessons of that time with a growing sense of urgency. Here are some ways to make do, mend and renew your things.

1. Change your shoes as often as you can.

Wearing the same pair of shoes day in, day out, makes them wear faster because they haven't been able to dry out from your feet's perspiration. When you get home, take off your shoes and have a pair of home shoes or slippers at the ready.

2. Drain, don't dry

Leave all the washing up, particularly china, to drain instead of drying it, to save wear on your tea towels.

3. Protect your hems

Sew a piece of hemming tape or old piece of material inside the bottom of each trouser leg where your shoes or boots rub, to prevent them from wearing thin.

4. Save those old scraps and slivers of soap.

When you have about 250–300 g worth, grate the soap scraps into a container, with a few drops of your favourite essential oil and just enough water for the shavings to clump together. Mould with your hands into new oval shapes and leave to dry for a couple of days before use.

5. Upcycle your skirt

An old skirt will make a little play-skirt and pair of bloomers for a toddler or young child. Consider mixing and matching a couple of different contrasting fabrics for a fun effect.

6. Secure your gloves

Wear gloves only to keep warm and, when you take them off, put them into your pocket or bag. Thousands of gloves are lost every year.

7. Swap your sleeves

If the sleeves of a hand-knit jumper or cardigan begin to wear on the underside and elbow, you can unpick and change them over to the opposite arms. This levels up the area of wear. (It's a good plan to damp-press them first to get rid of elbow bag.)

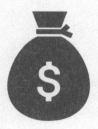

Whatever job you decide to do for work, no matter what it is, do to the best of your ability.

'This was advice given to me by Mother when I was deciding what to do for work when I was 14 years old.' – *Col Cotterill*

Don't wait until your last day of work to think about funding your retirement. Talk to a financial planner about how much money you need, and the best ways of topping up your superannuation to get there.

8 money-saving tips
that really work

1. Turn off appliances at the wall

You'd be surprised at how much energy is wasted by idle devices around the home. Standby power can contribute to as much as 10 per cent of your energy bill! Switch off that TV, stereo system and gaming console at the wall when you finish using them.

2. Selective toilet flushing

The old 'if it's yellow, let it mellow' rule may be derided by many, but if you're really looking to save a couple of dollars (and thousands of litres of water annually!), selective toilet flushing can be a good way to save.

3. Go cash only

Before you head to the shops, or once a week, withdraw the amount of money you wish to spend in cash. This way, you'll be much less likely to be tempted by those impulse buys and discretionary purchases.

4. Reuse disposable items

Depending on what you're storing in them, disposable items such as aluminium foil, zip-lock bags and fast-food containers can easily be used again and again.

5. Hit the hay earlier

Getting more shut-eye and waking up earlier takes advantage of daylight hours (which is free, by the way) and means you'll use less electricity during the evening.

6. Be a fiend for specials

Keep your ear to the ground and sign up for coupons, offers and specials that can help you do the things you'd normally do in day-to-day life, for much, much less.

7. Take a month off from a vice

Smoking and drinking aren't doing your health any good, and they're not helping your budget either. Taking a month off from a vice might be tricky, but your health and finances will thank you.

8. Make it a competition

Nothing drives effectiveness like the good-old competitive spirit. Start a friendly competition with family or friends to see who can save the most money over a given week or month.

Index

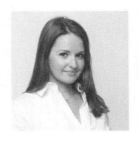

From age-old baking secrets to time-tested tips and tricks for a clean (and happy) home, Alexandra O'Brien's love of keeping traditions alive started at a young age, when she first remembers her grandmother, Patricia, cooking, sewing, entertaining and sharing her stories and wisdom with her grandchildren.

It was Alex's time writing at Over60 when, together with the team, they made it their mission to document stories and pearls of wisdom passed down for generations from mothers and grandmothers.

Reading these stories on the Over60 website each day it is clear how much joy the community find in being nostalgic and sharing tales from days gone. This book houses all of that passion in one handy manual so it can be cherished by generations to come.

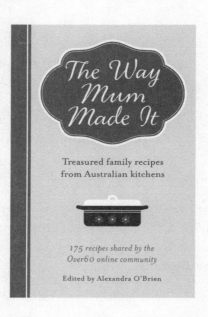

The Way Mum Made It

Treasured family recipes
from Australian kitchens

*175 recipes shared by the
Over60 online community*

Edited by Alexandra O'Brien

**Delicious recipes that are simple to
make, fuss-free and full of flavour.**

From the team behind the popular online community Over60
comes a cookbook featuring a collection of tried-and-true
favourites that have been passed down from
mother to daughter for generations.

With dishes to suit people living on their own as well as larger
families, there are chapters on breakfasts and brunches, sweet
treats for morning or afternoon tea, simple recipes that can
be made with the kids, easy lunches, delicious dinners, special
recipes for celebrations, as well as sauces, preserves and jams.
From old classics, like Mum's Sweet Brisket and The Perfect
Scones, to recipes with a modern twist, like Lemon and
Chicken Parmesan Rissoles and Raspberry Banana Bread
with Passionfruit Icing, there's something to
please every member of the family.

The perfect cookbook for anyone who appreciates
gathering around the table with loved ones to share
great food, with minimal effort.

Recipes from
The Way Mum Made It

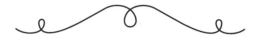

Banana split toasted sandwich

Perfect for breakfast, lunch or treat time, this old-school favourite can also be made to take out and about for a meal-on-the-run.

SERVES: 1

30 g butter
2 slices bread

50 g chocolate hazelnut spread
½ banana, sliced

1. Preheat the sandwich press or jaffle to medium–high heat. Butter one side of the two slices of bread.

2. Spread the chocolate hazelnut spread on both of the non-buttered sides of the bread. Layer the banana slices on the hazelnut spread side of one of the slices of bread. Place the other slice on top, with the buttered side facing up.

3. Grill the sandwich for 3 minutes, or until toasted. Cut the sandwich in half and serve immediately.

Parmesan-crusted baked chicken nuggets

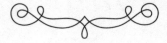

This recipe is great to make if you're having the grandkids over for dinner.
In fact, why not get them in the kitchen making this dish themselves?

SERVES: 4

500 g chicken breast fillets
1¼ cups garlic breadcrumbs
⅓ cup grated parmesan cheese
¼ teaspoon salt

1 tablespoon vegetable oil
4 tablespoons plain flour
2 large eggs, lightly beaten

1. Preheat the oven to 200°C. Cut the chicken into nugget-sized pieces.

2. Spread a thin layer of breadcrumbs on a baking tray and bake for 5 minutes, or until lightly golden.

3. Pour the breadcrumbs into a bowl with the parmesan and salt, and mix with the vegetable oil.

4. In small batches, coat the chicken pieces in the flour, shaking off any excess. Then dip in the beaten egg, before coating in the breadcrumbs.

5. Place on a lightly greased wire rack on top of a baking tray in the oven. Bake at 230°C for 10–12 minutes, turning halfway. Serve warm with your favourite dipping sauce.

    Note: To make this for one person, divide ingredients by four.

Kiss biscuits

*'My auntie, Edna McDermott, won first prize at the State
Cooking Contest in July 1976 with this kiss biscuit recipe. She
handwrote the recipe out for me about 30 years ago and it's still
very popular in our family. I am a third-generation member of
the Glenorchy Branch of the CWA of Tasmania.' Judith Morris*

MAKES: APPROXIMATELY 60

225 g self-raising flour
1 tablespoon cornflour
pinch of salt
110 g margarine (I use half
   unsalted butter and half
   margarine)

115 g sugar
1 egg
1 teaspoon vanilla extract

1. Preheat the oven to 180°C. Line a baking tray with baking
   paper.

2. Sift the flour, cornflour and salt into a bowl.

3. Using an electric mixer, cream the margarine and sugar.
   Add the egg and vanilla to the sugar mixture and beat well.

4. Add the flours gradually and mix until a soft dough forms.
   Roll out thinly and cut into rounds using a biscuit cutter.

5. Bake until lightly golden.